FIRST AID MANUAL

2023-2024

FIRST AID BOOK FOR TREATMENT AND PREVENTION OF ANY MEDICAL EMERGENCY WHEN YOU ARE OFF GRID

Dr. Allan Johnson

TABLE OF CONTENTS

INTRODUCTION

If you are hurt at home, knowing that help is only a 911 call away is both reassuring and perhaps lifesaving. Accidents may happen everywhere, but in the woods, a little injury can swiftly escalate into a big concern. When you are put into such a position, the game plan for emergency assistance has abruptly shifted, and you are completely on your own. What you must do now must be done sensibly if you or another injured person are to live.

Because there are no books, films, or articles that will instantaneously turn anyone become a physician, I wrote this book to serve as a reference to fundamental injuries, with a focus on preventative care. After reading this book, you should have a better concept of what steps to take to avoid getting into a disastrous scenario, especially in a remote setting where there is no medical facility.

If something happens to you or a partner in such a location, you may make a difference by providing competent, knowledgeable treatment using basic first-aid knowledge. These first-aid suggestions can help you stabilize diverse circumstances until experienced medical specialists can arrive to intervene and take care to the next level.

As someone who has spent a lot of time in remote areas, I would also advise anyone thinking about going to a place where medical care is limited or nonexistent to consult with their family doctor about medications, health precautions, vaccines, or whatever medical advice your doctor recommends to keep you healthy. After all, a good family physician knows his patient the best and can thus provide the finest recommendations.

Also, if you are a hunter or prefer guided wilderness adventures, you are well aware that going on a large game hunt or picture safari costs a lot of money. You are generally older and maybe out of shape by the time sufficient money is available. When choosing an outfitter or guide, look for someone who is a competent hunter and outdoorsman who is qualified in CPR and first aid.

When making a reservation, inquire about emergency care choices and their availability in his camp. Look for an experienced outfitter who understands that if a customer is not 21 and tough as nails, he must adapt the hunting tactics or travel mode to avoid pushing that first-time big game hunter or wilderness explorer over the brink. When many of us look in the mirror, it is clear that we are no longer the kids we once were, and tactical changes are necessary to avoid harm and stay healthy.

Unless a huge error is committed, the world of the outdoors is lovely and relatively safe. This is frequently the result of ignoring warning indicators of approaching peril. I'm not talking about grizzly bears or an impending avalanche, but rather the warning signs in your body that may suggest it's time for a check-up. It is up to you to be informed to the point where you can plan ahead and take the required measures to avoid harm or disease. If you plan ahead of time for the "what ifs," you will know what to do if something does happen. Remember, it is your responsibility to ensure your own health and safety.

A rudimentary understanding of first aid might be beneficial. It serves as a medical backup for prevention. The sooner you can avoid an injury or accident, the better. If something goes wrong, knowing basic first aid can save your life. However, keep in mind that doing anything that puts an injured person in greater danger may be worse than doing nothing. "Not harm!" is a medical adage.

Over the years, I've noticed that when a person is confronted with a disaster and does not panic, they'd be shocked at what can be achieved with basic information and a calm head. Developing this level of proficiency necessitates a combination of fundamental knowledge and common sense.

This is why planning for such circumstances, carrying basic emergency equipment, and knowing how to utilize it provide you with the skills you need to help yourself and others. With this information, you may enjoy hunting, hiking, and other outdoor activities safely!

Top Ten Emergency Response Procedures

1. Call 911 OR yell for help until you are certain that someone has heard you and contacted 911 OR go for help (either you OR someone else needs to call 911).

2. Assess the situation, ensure safety before proceeding, and keep your cool.

3. Check under ABCs and don't move anybody until absolutely required. Inquire with the individual who was injured about what happened.

4. If you have CPR training, do the Heimlich maneuver, and begin rescue breathing if someone is choking or having difficulty breathing. If the individual is not breathing or has no pulse, begin CPR.

5. Apply direct, consistent pressure to any bleeding areas.

6. Act swiftly if the individual feels clammy, pale, out of breath, chilly, or out of breath.

7. Examine any medical history or special needs for a medical alert bracelet, necklace, or identification tag (ORID card or driver's license).

8. Get professional medical aid when the injured individual has been stabilized.

9. Don't provide anything to sick or injured persons, including medications.

10. Wait for the ambulance while you console the ill or injured individual.

Myths about First Aid

The purpose of this book is to expose you to emergency response and basic first-aid techniques. The first and most important step in first aid is to prevent future injury. The book goes into detail on the essential principles for action, but the list that follows swiftly debunks some of the most common first-aid myths.

1. Patting someone on the back may cause the object to move. Let the individual choke. If the patient is coughing or having difficulty breathing, do the Heimlich maneuver.

2. Never use a tourniquet on or cut the skin of a snake bite victim.
3. Sucking might spread the venom and introduce additional bacteria, while a tourniquet would prevent blood from flowing to the area.

4. Peeing on a jellyfish sting will not ease your pain.

5. Hyperventilation may result from breathing into a paper bag.

6. Drinking alcohol in chilly weather can simply cause hypothermia.

7. Avoid consuming alcohol if you have a toothache or any other form of pain.

8. Applying butter, Crisco, or any other kind of grease to burns should be avoided since it might trap heat, promote an infection, and leave scars.

9. If you put a raw steak on a black eye or other injury, the bacteria on the meat may infect the wound or the eye.

10. To avoid destroying the body's defense cells that are rushing to the site to cope with invading pathogens, avoid washing wounds with hydrogen peroxide.

11. People DO NOT swallow their tongues during seizures, so don't try to grasp your tongue or put anything in your mouth. Don't either.

12. Scrape the stinger off a stung bee using a credit card rather than squeezing or trying to remove it with tweezers, since this might suck poison into the wound.

13. Throwing your head back during a nosebleed may cause blood to run down your neck and perhaps cause you to vomit. Instead, take a little step forward and breathe through your nose for 10 minutes.

14. If the item has the potential to seal a cut and stop bleeding, you should not remove it. If you are doubtful, get medical help.

15. Running when injured can aggravate your shin splints, so avoid doing so.

16. Rather of vinegar, use COLD compresses on a sunburn.

17. You can't get rid of motion sickness by staring at a certain point in space.

18. The oil is communicable, but poison ivy is not. If the oil is on you, it may spread to others.

19. Avoid applying alcohol to a fever since it will penetrate the skin and potentially spread the illness.

Chapter 1

First Aid Basics

Since first aid is complex and situational, the more informed and skillful you are, the more ready you will be to deal with any unanticipated illness or disaster. When someone is hurt or becomes unexpectedly ill, the first thing you do is provide them first aid. But first aid entails more than simply having a well-stocked first-aid kit; it also entails being able to prevent, prepare for, detect, and swiftly treat small mishaps, as well as understanding what to do in an emergency. You can cure many common ailments and injuries if you know what to do. But you must first evaluate if first aid would adequate or whether expert help is required. Understanding how to react until help arrives may save a life when the situation requires efforts beyond basic first aid.

Stay Calm

Being prepared is the best way to prevent panic. Being ready for anything allows you to stay calm, analyze the situation quickly, and take more effective action. Being structured allows you to be collected and confident, which will help the injured person feel more at ease. To be prepared, post emergency phone numbers near the phones at your house and place of work. In addition to 911, key numbers to keep on hand are the fire department, the nearest hospital, the Poison Control Center (1-800-222-1222), and your family doctor. Urge family members with serious medical issues to wear a medical alert tag or bracelet and have a list of their medical conditions and emergency phone numbers on hand. Moreover, rehearse your home escape strategy with your children. Keep a fire extinguisher on hand and teach every member of your home how to use it.

CAUTION!

Owing to the potential dangers of many first-aid supplies, it is critical to keep them away from children and pets. Your kit should be placed in a spot that is both accessible and out of reach for a child or pet, either on their own or with the assistance of a chair, for example.

The Right Supplies

To provide proper first aid, you will need a decent first-aid kit. The better stocked and organized your first-aid kit is, the faster you can respond to events in your house. Have a written inventory of your kit's components at your house, in addition to your emergency plan. Replace anything with an open box or a broken seal that is meant to be sterile and refill the kit as needed. In your emergency kit, include a first aid manual like this one, a list of emergency phone numbers, a synopsis of your family's medical problems and medicines, and a flashlight.

NOTE!

Your local pharmacy or doctor's office may be able to offer you with Medic Alert identification. On these jewelry identification tags, your critical medical conditions (such as allergies), ID number, and 24-hour emergency response center number are often imprinted.

A Proper Container

Make sure it's clearly labeled "First-Aid Kit," and select a container with a solid handle that can be tightly clamped shut. Commercial kits are available from several places, but a large, robust plastic fishing-tackle box may do the job just as well and is typically much less costly.

The perfect kit should be compact enough to store all necessary items in an orderly and accessible manner, but light enough to carry. It must be water and dust resistant, as well as sturdy enough to endure crushing or falling.

How to Store your Equipment

Maintain your equipment in a cool, dry area of your home. Because of the dangers that change in moisture and temperature bring to its contents, avoid keeping it in the garage or laundry room. Pick a spot in your house that is accessible and handy for everyone who will be using the kit.

The Ideal Kit

The following items should be included in the ideal kit to protect you from many accidents and domestic emergencies:

- Antacid (liquid)
- Activated charcoal (only use if instructed by the Poi-son Control Center)
- Antibiotic ointment or cream
- Benadryl (generic Diphenhydramine)
- Povidone-iodine solution
- 1% hydrocortisone cream
- Antihistamine cream
- Calamine lotion
- Extra prescribed medications (such as inhalers)
- Epinephrine auto-injector kit (if prescribed by your doctor)
- Sterile eye-wash solution
- Aspirin, ibuprofen, and acetaminophen

The following bandages and dressing supplies should be included in your emergency kit:

- Sterile gauze (pads and rolls)
- Cotton-tipped swabs
- Sterile cotton balls
- Commercial band-aid bandages
- Sterile eye patches
- Butterfly bandages

- Extra bandage clips
- Extra bandage rolls
- Large foil-lined bandage
- Triangular bandages
- Adhesive tape (waterproof and elastic)
- Regular adhesive bandages (multiple sizes)

NOTE!
Epinephrine should only be used in extreme circumstances by persons having sudden, severe symptoms or reactions to any allergy, including foods, insect stings, and inhalation allergies. If anybody in your family has ever had this kind of reaction, ask your family doctor to prescribe an epinephrine auto-injector and give you with instructions on how to use it.

In addition, the following tools and other items should be included:

- Hand sanitizer
- Clean clothes and tissues
- Small paper cups
- Medicine spoon (transparent tube with standard pharmaceutical dosages inscribed on it)
- Bulb syringe
- Safety pins
- Disposable CPR face mask
- Sterile disposable gloves

- Small jar of petroleum jelly
- Digital thermometer (also a rectal thermometer for babies less than a year old)
- Penlight
- Space blanket
- Tooth-preservation kit
- Tweezers
- Scissors (the sharp, angular style with a rounded end)
- Whistle
- Magnifying glass
- Disposable self-activating packs (cold and hot)
- Emergency candle and waterproof matches
- Small notepad and pencil

> ***CAUTION!***
>
> *Children under the age of sixteen should never be given aspirin or children's aspirin if they have flu-like symptoms or chicken pox. Aspirin may cause Reye's syndrome, a potentially lethal illness affecting the liver and brain system.*

In putting together your pack, consider your family's medical history, including any drug allergies and risk factors. Furthermore, keep these medication warnings in mind. Even when used as directed, aspirin, ibuprofen, and other nonsteroidal anti-inflammatory drugs (NSAIDs) may cause kidney damage and gastrointestinal bleeding. Individuals over the age of 49, people with stomach ulcers, and anybody who takes blood-thinning medications or steroids while taking NSAIDs for an extended period are at a higher risk. There is a risk of significant liver damage when patients take more acetaminophen than is suggested or drink three or more alcoholic beverages while taking it. Read the labels of all drugs to verify that you are not exceeding the prescribed maximum dose of four grams or four thousand milligrams per day for a healthy adult. Acetaminophen is included in a variety of over the counter (OTC) drugs.

VITAL!

All information about your family that you, paramedics, or doctors may require for reference should be recorded on your family's medical list or chart, including shot records with dates, medical conditions and maladies, medications, and allergies.

Getting Medical Information

Our family's medical history is a complete collection of health information from three generations of relatives that helps physicians understand the different aspects that are common to our family, such as genes, environment, and lifestyle. This medical history may assist you in determining your risk of developing a condition, such as heart disease, high blood pressure, stroke, certain cancers, or diabetes, by providing information about medical conditions that may run in your family as well as specific patterns of disorders.

An information record should include a family member's full name, birth date, allergies, medical history, current and previous medications, immunization records, injury history, any disabilities, rehabilitations, addiction and substance abuse history and treatment, previous hospitalizations, and surgeries. Enter any contact information a first responder could require in the case of a disaster or in circumstances when someone might not be present to provide the information.

In your medical information record, include the names and contact information for your physicians, the amount of your insurance coverage, who to call in an emergency, and even your preferred religion.

Calling 911

You may be hesitant to call 911 if you are unclear if the medical condition or complaint is really an emergency due to fear, humiliation, or other issues.

There are several conditions that require immediate attention, so don't hesitate to dial 911. If you are unsure, it is best to seek help rather than risking serious consequences or even death. The following are scenarios that demand contacting 911, while this is by no means an exhaustive list:

- Severe allergic reaction
- Shortness of breath, heart attack, or chest pain
- Asthma attack or respiratory arrest

- Loss of consciousness or responsiveness
- Confusion, fainting, dizziness, or convulsions are all symptoms of convulsions.
- Chemical exposure, poisoning, or drug overdose
- Heat exhaustion
- Rectal bleeding, bloody diarrhea, bleeding when weakened, or vomiting blood.
- Stuttering, paralysis, or any other stroke symptoms
- Uncontrolled bleeding, such as nosebleeds
- Serious burns
- Broken bones with indications of head or spinal damage
- Suicidal behavior, self-harm, or violent behavior

CAUTION!

If you are experiencing any of the signs of a heart attack, dial 911. Immediately—there is a very short window of time before irreversible cardiac muscle damage develops. If you arrive by ambulance, you will get faster treatment at the hospital since emergency medical services (EMS) are trained to address cardiac arrest both on the scene and while you are in transit.

Unless you are using a mobile phone or calling from a site where phones are linked to a switchboard, the dispatcher's computer will most likely indicate your location. Keeping your cool will allow you to answer to questions as quickly and thoroughly as possible. All the information mentioned here will be required by the dispatcher.

- What is the emergency?
- When the crisis first began
- Location of the precise area where help is needed.
- What phone number are you dialing?
- Your name, as well as others, is mentioned.

Remain on the phone until the 911 dispatcher tells you to hang up, or until it is safe to do so, and follow all their instructions. Be calm, clear, and attentive to the dispatcher's instructions, and react as briefly as possible.

> ***VITAL!***
>
> *It is the 911 dispatcher's job to ask the required questions. Take your time and try your best to answer every question. Don't hang up until told; if you're on a mobile phone, you may need to give your exact location and other data since the dispatcher can't see where you are.*

Informing Children

To show young children how to dial 911, use a toy phone or an old, non-functioning mobile phone. Inform them that emergencies include car accidents, criminal acts such as causing injury or breaking into a property, when a family member gets suddenly terribly unwell (for example, having difficulties speaking or breathing or turning blue), if someone collides or passes out, or if the house is on fire.

> ***NOTE!***
>
> *Most children above the age of five are capable of grasping, learning, and knowing when to dial 911. Encourage children to only call 911 in actual emergencies. Assure children that when they phone 911, police and firemen will respond.*

.

Global Precautions

There is a danger of communicable sickness when doing first aid. In addition to following conventional safety protocols, you should use personal protection gear like as gloves, a CPR barrier, or eye protection (also known as universal precautions). When exposed to blood, bodily fluids (including sperm and vaginal fluid), and tissue from an infectious person, universal precautions protect caregivers against HIV (the virus that causes AIDS), hepatitis B, and other blood-borne infections.

All fluids, including amniotic (from a pregnant uterus), cerebrospinal (from the lining of the brain and spinal cord), synovial (from the joint), pleural (from the lung), peritoneal (from the belly), and pericardial, should be handled with care (from the heart). Saliva, urine, sweat, tears, nasal secretions, sputum, and feces are excluded from these guidelines unless they include blood. Professional general safety precautions include the following:

1. Wash your hands before and after obtaining medical assistance.

2. Use gloves whenever you come into touch with another person's blood, body fluids, or tissues, even if the person you're aiding is a family member.
3. Put on a face mask or body suit if the rescuer is likely to be sprayed with blood.
4. Sharp items that have been contaminated should be placed in a puncture-proof container.
5. Put all contaminated equipment in the appropriate biohazard container to be disposed of.
6. Even if you lack all the necessary equipment, these professional tips will guide you in the right direction. As a layman, you should try to follow these safety rules as strictly as possible.

CAUTION!

To protect your health and maybe save lives, take precautions anytime you encounter blood or other physiological fluids or secretions that may contain blood.

Even if you know the person well, you should use a protective barrier while providing care to them. Currently, it seems basic sense to avoid contact with an unknown cause of sickness. If you don't have any romantic connections, make do with something like plastic wrap. Additionally, before and after providing care, be sure to properly wash your hands.

The Right Training

Nothing can replace the practical training you get from formal instruction in a classroom environment, even while this book is intended to be a comprehensive resource that covers first-aid fundamentals. Anybody can study first aid, and by brushing up on old knowledge and learning new lifesaving techniques, you'll feel and behave more confident at home, at work, and while traveling.

Several organizations, including the American Red Cross, the American Heart Association, and the National Safety Association, provide first-aid training courses. Some local EMS organizations also offer Basic Life Support (BLS) courses. Most charge a minimal fee for a one- to two-day course on CPR and basic first aid; certain organizations sometimes provide free one-day seminars to the community.

VITAL!

Global precautions DO NOT indicate that you should not provide care; they just recommend that you be careful and avoid incurring risks.

Chapter 2

Emergency First Aid

To save lives, it is widely accepted that CPR should begin as soon as a person falls or has "witnessed arrest" (when someone sees the event Occur). Yet, in situations of witnessed arrest, only about a third of individuals or fewer respond, and even when CPR is started immediately, it is often performed improperly. As a result, it is essential to get CPR and AED certificates, as well as to complete the highly recommended refresher certification courses. In an emergency, learning CPR may help you save lives, decrease disability, enhance your health, and even reverse clinical death.

The History of CPR

In 1740, the Paris Academy of Sciences generally advised mouth-to-mouth resuscitation for near-drowning patients, which is where cardiopulmonary resuscitation (CPR) got its start. In 1891, Dr. Friedrich Maass conducted the first known and effective human chest compression. Rather of using external chest compressions in human resuscitation, it has been tested and confirmed throughout the years that a rescuer's exhaled air is sufficient to oxygenate an unconscious individual. Since CPR was fully created and deployed in 1960, the American Heart Association (AHA) gave CPR training and urged the general populace to utilize it. The American Red Cross and other organizations collaborated to develop performance standards, standardized teaching, and CPR certification for use in the treatment of acute, life-threatening cardiovascular disorders such as sudden cardiac arrest.

Every five years, the AHA guidelines for CPR and emergency cardiac care are assessed, improved, and amended to raise the survival rates of life-threatening situations. AHA creates these guidelines with the help of other organizations, peer-reviewed research, and other systematic evidence-based analysis and assessment. This page provides a summary of the most recent AHA CPR and resuscitation protocol from 2005.

The ABCs of First Aid

There are three critical steps in emergency first aid. To live, a human need both basic life support and all three common denominators. ORCPR and early defibrillation have been demonstrated to improve long-term survival following a cardiac arrest. This book gives an overview of basic cardiac resuscitation procedures, but it should not be used in place of proper training or exercises. It should be used as an introduction instead. To find out where to take CPR and first aid classes, contact the American Red Cross or the American Heart Association.

The ABCs of circulation, breathing, and airway are the abbreviations for first aid:

- **Airway:** Is the airway clear to breathe? Take steps to clear the airway.
- **Breathing:** Does the individual seem to be breathing? Start your rescue breathing now.
- **Circulation:** Is the subject's heart beating? Begin the chest compressions.

CPR and AED Basics

According to the American Heart Association, doing CPR involves a series of assessments and actions. Moreover, since cardiac arrest is not caused by a single problem, the phases of CPR will vary based on the kind or cause of the event. For the purposes of this book, only lay rescuer strategies and approaches will be addressed. It's vital to remember that lay rescuers are no longer advised to check for pulse, signs of circulation, or to offer rescue breathing to an unconscious individual without doing chest compressions. When you witness someone above the age of one fall, do the following steps:

1. Check to see whether approaching the individual who has fallen is safe.
2. Use safety equipment and take standard precautions. Utilize common sense and avoid any evident hazards as much as possible.
3. To rouse the individual, rub their sternum (breastbone) with your knuckles while yelling, "Are you okay?"

4. If the victim is unable to awaken, call 911 immediately. Depending on your situation, get help. Furthermore, if an AED is close, request that someone bring it to you.
5. If the victim becomes cognizant, moans, or moves, DO NOT start CPR.
6. Dial 911 if the individual is unable to converse or seems disoriented. If the victim does not wake up, begin CPR, and use an AED if one is available.

An AED, a small, portable electronic device, is used to shock the heart with electricity to halt or interrupt abnormal electrical activity. A continuously aberrant rhythm is inadequate to pump blood and deliver oxygen throughout the body. An AED shock cannot restore a dead heart, it must be beating (even though the rhythm is abnormal). If leads are linked to an unconscious individual, the AED will detect any cardiac arrhythmia automatically. When one of these dangerous rhythms is found, you may use an AED or a shock (defibrillation) to terminate the arrhythmia and enable the heart to return to a healthy and productive rhythm. You may learn how to use an AED in a variety of first aid, first-responder, and CPR classes.

VITAL!

The American Heart Association urges rescuers to utilize maximal force, apply force fast (100 compressions per minute), allow complete chest recoil between compressions, and stop compressions as little as possible for all patients.

Follow these steps while doing CPR:

1. To open the airway, use the head-tilt, chin-lift method. Put one hand on the forehead and the fingers of the other hand towards the chin under the bony region of the lower jaw. Tilt the head back, taking careful not to pinch the mouth or push on sensitive tissues beneath the chin, to gradually lift the jaw. If you have spinal injury, avoid lifting your neck.

2. Listen for air going through the mouth or nose, angle your head to see the person's chest movement, and feel for breath on your cheek to determine if they are breathing properly. A person who sometimes gasps is most likely having a heart attack and needs CPR.

3. If there are no signs of breathing, pinch the nose to create a seal. Give the individual a forceful enough breath so you can see the chest rise over the mouth with yours. If the chest descends, repeat the rescue breath. Once again, for a total of two breaths. Place a CPR mask between your lips and the person you're rescuing if one is available. The first three steps are referred to be "rescue breathing."

4. To begin chest compressions, lay your palm's heel on the bottom portion of your breastbone around the nipple line in the middle of your chest. Link your fingers together and press your chest forward by one to two inches with the heel of one hand on the chest and the heel of the other hand on the top of that hand. Let the chest to fully retract before delivering thirty 100-pressure-per-minute pressures.

5. After thirty chest compressions, immediately repeat the two rescue breaths. To broaden your airway, tilt your head back and lift your chin. This time, instead of checking for breathing, go straight to rescue breaths. Breathe in one, making sure your chest rises and falls, and then exhale.

6. Do the cycle of thirty contractions followed by two breaths for roughly two minutes. Next, come to a halt and double-check your breathing. If the individual is not breathing, continue chest compressions and rescue breathing.

Other Applications

The American Heart Association (AHA) presently recommends that everyone, regardless of age, do a set of thirty compressions followed by two breaths (a compression-ventilation ratio of 30:2). Continue the cycle of compressions and rescue breathing until skilled help arrives or the individual begins to breathe on their own. With youngsters aged one to eight, use one or two hands to squeeze the chest one-third to one-half its depth. For the unresponsive infant or child, do five cycles of thirty compressions and two breaths for around two minutes before leaving the child to call 911 and get an AED if one is available.

CPR for Babies and Infants

The guidelines for neonatal CPR differ from those for infants. However, newborn CPR guidelines only apply to newborns in the initial hours after birth until the baby leaves the hospital, therefore the public should only be concerned with infant CPR recommendations that apply to babies less than roughly one year of age. The rescue breathing rate for babies with pulses is roughly 40 to 60 breaths per minute, with chest compression to a depth of one-third of the chest. Every minute, do 30 ventilations and 90 compressions. Compress the infant's chest with two fingers just below the nipple line (on the lower half of the sternum) for a compression-ventilation ratio of 30:2.

Problems with CPR

The AHA has discovered many difficulties with CPR performance, including excessive breathing during CPR and compressions that are often interrupted, too slowly, and too slowly. According to hypothesis, bystanders may be unwilling to perform CPR because they find it too intricate and difficult to remember. In recent modifications, the AHA has attempted to expedite processes by adopting the same compression-ventilation ratio for infants, children, and adults. The identical adjustment has been made for both adult and child chest imprints.

While the statistics suggest that the risk of infection transmission is very minimal, using a barrier device (CPR mask) when doing ventilations is still recommended. It has been proposed that the general population is fearful of getting infections and, therefore, is hesitant to do mouth-to-mouth resuscitation. Even if you are still afraid to do mouth-to-mouth ventilations, seek for help and begin chest compressions as soon as possible.

CAUTION!

If you or a family member already has a cardiac problem or is at high risk of heart failure, your doctor may be able to prescribe an AED that is at least partially covered by your medical plan.

Recovery Position

The recovery position is used as first aid for all unconscious patients who are breathing. This category includes anyone over the age of one who has resumed breathing after receiving CPR, those who may be unconscious or nearly unconscious but are still breathing, those who are too inebriated to ensure they are still breathing, those who have come dangerously close to drowning, and those suspected of being poisoned.

A person who is unconscious and lying face up may have an airway obstruction. When laying face up, the tongue may relax towards the back of the throat, where body fluids such as blood or vomit may pool and obstruct the airway. When someone is face-up, the esophagus is slightly tilted downward from the stomach toward the neck, and this, combined with the loss of muscle control that occurs when someone is unconscious, may result in passive regurgitation, or when the contents of the stomach flow up into the throat. Aside from airway Obstruction, any fluid collecting at the back of the throat may flow down into the lungs, where the acid from the stomach can harm the lungs, a condition known as aspiration pneumonia.

The original injury or illness that knocked someone out of consciousness may not be fatal in many situations, but the passive regurgitation or aspiration pneumonia that comes from it generally is.

Excessive alcohol intake, which causes loss of consciousness and is followed by all OR some of these events, is a leading cause of mortality. When in an upright position, gravity prevents fluids from flowing in the wrong direction and keeps the tongue from obstructing the airway. When combined with lifting the chest off the ground, this helps to shield the person while also facilitating respiration.

> ***VITAL!***
>
> *If someone is unconscious after an accident, fall, collision, or other trauma, you must presume they have spinal injuries and take care to support the neck.*

As with any first aid scenario, assess the surroundings for safety before approaching the unconscious person. Then, assess the person for the ABCs. If there is no need for CPR or if you have already performed it and the individual begins breathing, place them in the recovery position. If there is no sign of spinal or neck damage, the individual should be in the lateral recovery position:

1. Kneel to one side and face the individual on his back with your legs outstretched. Position the person's arm closest to

you perpendicular to his body, elbow flexed. The hand should then be positioned across the body while the opposite arm is in place.

2. Pull the thigh towards you by reaching behind the knee of the leg farthest away from you.
3. Roll the body toward you while tugging the furthest distant shoulder with your other arm. Keep the upper leg flexed to help stabilize the body.

If emergency assistance is delayed, you may rotate the individual from side to side once every thirty minutes since persons who stay in this position for an extended period may develop nerve compression. Any movement of the unbalanced neck after a spinal injury increases the risk of permanent paralysis or other consequences, thus movement should be limited. The sole purpose to shift someone with a suspected spinal injury into a recovery position is to clear the airway of vomit. You should then use the HAINES modified recovery position (High Arm IN Endangered Spine). Turn the wounded person's body to support the head and neck for pain-free neck mobility, while lifting one of the injured person's damaged arms above the head (in full abduction).

When there is a suspected spine or neck injury, the primary priority is to keep the airway open. If the individual is still alive, leave them where you found them. Yet, if breathing stops, you must continue with ABCs: airway, breathing, and circulation, regardless of the possibility of additional harm to the person. All else comes second to breathing.

A pregnant woman who is unconscious should always be placed on her left side, and anyone with extremity injuries should be placed so that the wounds are closest to the ground to reduce the risk of blood oozing into the lungs.

An infant under a year old should be put in a modified recovery position, which involves being held in the arms with the head leaned down to prevent airway blockage or vomit inhalation. Continue to monitor the person's level of responsiveness, pulse, and breathing until help arrives.

Warning Signs of a Heart Attack

While heart attacks are uncommon, they may happen quickly and without warning. Most heart attacks begin slowly, with just little pain. The greatest mistake is when individuals wait far too long to seek aid because they are apprehensive. If you or someone you know is suffering any of the following symptoms, get help immediately away:

- Unbearable pressure, squeezing, fullness, or pain that comes and goes in the center of the chest for more than a few minutes are examples of chest discomfort.
- Discomfort in other upper body areas, such as the back, neck, jaw, or stomach, or pain in one OR both arms
- Shortness of breath

- Sweating, dizziness, or nausea

Other typical symptoms, such as back or jaw pain, shortness of breath, nausea, and vomiting, are more prevalent in women. Even if you are hesitant, it is best to contact 911. If you are unable to get Emergency Medical Services, have someone else bring you to the hospital as soon as possible (EMS). Only drive when there are no other choices.

QUESTION?

Do men and women have heart attacks the same way?

Women are more prone than men to have back or jaw pain, shortness of breath, nausea, and vomiting. A doctor should treat all symptoms, not only the "classic" heart attack symptoms, very soon.

What is going on?

The heart works mechanically as well as electrically. When it takes blood, you may feel a pulse, which is how it pumps blood—its mechanical function. The heart also contains cells that trigger muscle tissue to contract (the electrical function) by transmitting electrical impulses via conduction routes. During rest, the frequency of electrical stimulation or pulses should be between sixty and eighty times per minute, increasing with exertion. It should be connected to the frequency of cardiac muscle contractions or beats in general.

The ventricles are the heart's pumping chambers. SCA develops when the heart suddenly stops drawing and pumping blood into the body. Ventricular fibrillation (VF) is a disorganized and abnormal rhythm and spasmodic twitching of the heart that prevents it from adequately pumping blood throughout the body. A person in VF ORV fib typically has no pulse when the heart isn't pumping blood. They go unconscious, cease breathing, and die within minutes if not treated.

Choking

When something gets trapped in the throat and partly or fully closes the airway, it causes choking. Checking indicators include:

- Pointing to the throat / hands crossed on throat (universal sign of choking)
- Gasping or coughing
- Indications of anxiety
- Difficulty in speaking
- A red face that gradually turns blue
- Loss of Consciousness

CAUTION!

Never hit the back of someone you fear is choking. When a baby is crying, seems to be breathing normally, and has a severe cough, it should be seated up and allowed time to cough. Never attempt to remove an object from someone who is coughing by shoving your fingers down their throat, whether it is a baby or another person.

"Are you choking?" ask the individual you suspect of choking. If the individual can reply to you, don't take any action since she will most likely release the food or object on her own. You will need to support the individual in the case of actual talking since they will be unable to speak. If the individual is unable to talk, make noises, breathe adequately, or is unconscious, call 911 before doing the Heimlich maneuver, as seen below. If the victim is unconscious, place them on her back. Check the person's mouth for visible impediments and try to remove them with a finger sweep. If you are unable to do so, begin mouth-to-mouth resuscitation and CPR. Continue to check inside the person's mouth for any indicators of the foreign body as the chest compressions OF CPR may dislodge it.

The Heimlich Maneuver

The Heimlich maneuver, pronounced "Hi-mlick," involves giving abdominal thrusts to oneself or the individual who is strangled. The Heimlich maneuver should not be used on newborns under one year old; rather, it should be used on cognizant adults and children above the age of one to release a clogged airway. An abdominal thrust, like coughing, lifts the diaphragm and drives air out of the lungs to move and clear foreign materials in an airway.

On a coughing individual, do the Heimlich maneuver as follows:

1. Move behind the individual, wrap your arms around the waist, and lean them gently forward.

2. Make a fist with one hand and place it right over the navel.
3. Apply force as if you were attempting to drag the individual off the ground by pushing your fist forcefully into the abdomen while gripping it with your other hand.
4. Continue thrusting until the foreign body has been moved.

If you are choking, the steps to do the Heimlich maneuver on yourself are as follows:

1. Form a fist and put it over your navel.
2. Bend over any hard surface, such as a chair or counter, with your other hand gripping your fist and press your fist upward and inward.

To clear an airway blockage in an obese or pregnant person, place your hands close to your chest, just above the rib junction at the base of the breastbone, and do the Heimlich maneuver. When she is choking, lower the unconscious person on her back to the floor. To open the airway, use the head-tilt technique. If you can see the debris, reach into the mouth, and sweep it out (finger sweep), being cautious not to push the item farther into the airway. If you are unable to remove the obstructing item and the person does not respond, you must begin CPR. In this case, the chest compressions used during CPR may cause the item to be released, necessitating frequent examination of the mouth.

If you have a choking infant over the age of one, sit with the kid face down on your forearm, securely positioned on your thigh. Gently but strongly pound the infant five times with the heel of your hand in the center of the back. The back bends and gravity will most likely relieve the impediment. If it doesn't work, try flipping the baby face up on your forearm, head lower than body. Then, rapidly press the baby's chest five times with two fingers positioned over the breastbone right below the nipples. Continue the back blows and chest thrusts as needed and call 911 if the infant is still not breathing. Start neonatal CPR if the impediment has been removed but the infant is still not breathing. Only provide abdominal thrusts to babies above the age of one year.

NOTE!

Unintentional injuries from accidents such as motor vehicle collisions, chokings, and suffocations, near drownings, bicycle-related wrecks, falls, and poisonings are the leading causes of death for children aged fourteen and younger. Being educated in CPR and first aid might save a child's life!

Swallowing Strange Objects

Children and adults in altered states caused by disorders such as stroke and alcohol misuse, as well as people who wear dentures, are more susceptible than others to swallow tiny foreign items unknowingly. Coins and batteries which are widespread in households and are often swallowed by foreign items, should be kept out of children's reach. Denture wearers must take additional measures since they lack the touch feeling in their mouths, which might protect them from eating items such as bones. Foreign objects may get stuck in the esophagus (swallowing pathway) and cause symptoms such as drooling and retching, chest pain, choking, and swallowing difficulty. Within a few hours, other symptoms such as vomiting, nausea, stomach discomfort, blood in the stool, and fever may occur.

First Aid for Swallowing a Strange Object

Do the Heimlich maneuver as outlined in detail for anybody experiencing signs of an airway blockage. Some people with chronic symptoms should seek medical attention, since in 20% of cases, the object must be removed by a doctor using an endoscope procedure. Batteries deteriorate and produce chemicals that may cause significant injury, thus any child suspected of possessing a battery should be sent to the emergency department straight once. Other non-caustic things often pass through on their own once the initial effort has faded. If you have any questions or concerns, always seek the counsel of a health care practitioner.

Managing Shock

Controlling and avoiding shock is critical in an emergency. Shock occurs when the circulatory system fails to transfer blood to the body. Shock may occur when the heart beats irregularly, blood vessels dilate rapidly, or a person loses an excessive quantity of blood. Shock symptoms include a weak and rapid pulse, disorientation, dizziness, faintness, cold, clammy hands and skin, extreme thirst, nausea, and vomiting, as well as a high level of anxiety and fingernails that DO NOT blanch when pressure is applied (turn white when pressed and color does not return within two seconds).

You must safeguard the victim from shock in an emergency. Since you cannot manage the person's shock alone and they are likely to fall into cardiac arrest, contact 911 immediately. While waiting for help, keep checking the ABCs and, if required, begin CPR. If the head, neck, back, hips, or legs are not harmed, place the person face up on the ground and raise the legs to keep vital blood flowing to vital organs. To stop bleeding, apply pressure to open wounds using a towel, sanitary napkin, or piece of clothing. Regardless of whether the person claims to be thirsty, never offer them water; instead, keep them quiet, comfortable, and warm. Until help arrives, keep reminding the person of the ABCs and their natural curiosity.

Chapter 3

Preventive First Aid

Accidents are the leading cause of adult injuries and the most common location for injuries and acute illnesses to occur. Preventative measures are critical since it has been shown that human error is the main cause of most accidents. This chapter will help keep you and your family safer at home by outlining the preventive measures you should take.

Taking Safety Measures

It is still true that "an ounce of prevention is worth a pound of cure," since it is considerably easier to spend a little effort avoiding disasters than coping with them. Examine your surroundings for potential hazards and unsafe activities. Assess what you can do to remove these danger zones, and then implement the necessary safety and preventive measures.

Toxins

Toxins in cosmetics may harm the skin and enter via damaged skin. Working with potentially hazardous items and anything with a warning label requires the use of protective gloves and clothing because others are absorbed even if they DO NOT cause skin injury. Even if you wear glasses, several chemical compounds are highly hazardous to your eyes and should be used with protective goggles.

Goggles are available at a variety of drugstores and home improvement shops.

CAUTION!

The phrase "nontoxic" refers to a medicine that has little to no harmful effects when taken or breathed. It does not guarantee that the product is safe. Note that any product you've used that contains chemicals might be the source of any illness or bad reaction.

You can determine if a product is one you want in your house by reading the label and directions, which will also tell you how to use it and what to do in the case of an emergency involving ingestion or contact with the eyes. Products with the words "Caution," "Poison," "Danger," or "Warning" on the label should be avoided.

Proper ventilation, as well as the use of fans and open windows, is essential when using any kind of aerosol or volatile poison. This is because anything circulating in the air will enter the circulation via our lungs. If you can smell it, we need to enhance our ventilation. Using a mask is a good suggestion for our personal protection since certain dangerous materials have no scents.

VITAL!

Never mix things unless the maker clearly states that it is okay to do so. Product combinations may result in explosive or deadly chemical reactions.

Read and then follow the instructions! Keep a tight seal on all lids and follow the manufacturer's storage instructions. Whenever possible, work outdoors or take regular breaks to obtain some fresh air. If you begin to feel lightheaded, queasy, or headachy, take a break, walk outdoors, or even stop working entirely.

For pests, baits, and traps are the safest pesticides because they DO NOT make the whole area you are treating hazardous and are designed so that the pest enters the container carrying the poison and then returns it to the colony nest.

Alternatives to insecticides include insecticidal soaps, beneficial nematodes (good bugs that eat the pesty Ones), neem oil (a natural insecticide), diatomaceous earth (not the swimming-pool variety), B.T., microbial insecticides, beneficial nematodes, insecticidal soaps, frequent vacuuming, and beneficial nematodes. Try enzyme sprays, spraying the pet with a 50:50 mix of white vinegar and water, washing the pet's bedding once a week, and regular vacuuming for flea management.

Items should be kept away from corrosive elements, in their original containers with the original labels still attached, and combustible goods should be stored separately. When working with flammable compounds like furniture stripper or paint remover, keep rags in a sealed, labeled container, preferably made of metal, away from heat or ignition sources that might set them fire.

NOTE!

If you are pregnant, avoid being exposed to hazardous chemicals since many deadly items have either never been tested to determine whether they would harm an unborn baby or have been developed, sold, and then shown to be toxic and withdrawn from the market.

Safety from Fire

The US Fire Administration recommends placing functional smoke detectors in every bedroom, in rooms other than the bedroom, and on each level of your house. They also recommend that you examine your smoke detectors every week, update the batteries once a year, and replace them 10 years after you first use them. Since flames only travel upstairs, you should have escape ladders to help you get out of a house's second story and practice using them while practicing your escape plan. Never try to put out an unmanageable fire; instead, make a quick retreat and seek help. Thus have an ABC ORABCD fire extinguisher on available and learn how to use it in the event of a little, controlled fire in the kitchen, garage, or office.

VITAL!

Smoke detectors will allow you to escape in the case of a fire, but you should also establish and practice an emergency evacuation strategy with two exit routes from each room. Arrange an outside gathering spot for the family once they've evacuated.

Keep screens clean and fireplaces clean. A professional cleaning of chimneys and stovepipes once a year is suggested to avoid creosote, which may catch fire and cause a home fire.

Safety in the Kitchen

When a pot of liquid or other object is left unattended and begins to burn, this is the most frequent kind of kitchen fire. When anything greasy catches fire while cooking, it may spark open flames that soon evolve into a destructive inferno, which is how grease fires originate. To put out a kitchen fire, follow these steps:

- Turn off the stove, if possible.
- If a pan is on fire and a lid can be used to put it out, do so.
- Never use water to put out a grease fire or take a flaming pan outside or to the sink.
- Keep a fire blanket in your kitchen so you can gently toss it over a fire while covering your hands.
- Set timers to remind you of the food you are cooking even if you believe you will remember.
- Dish towels, bags, and other flammable materials should be kept away from the stove.
- Never use dish towels to handle hot pots, pans, and baking trays; instead, use potholders or oven mitts.

Making Your Home Childproof

When you have a kid, you should totally commit to attending seminars and readings on how to keep your child safe at home. The guidelines that follow will provide you a broad overview of how to childproof your house.

Physical Dangers

Electrical outlets are sometimes intriguing to children. Several are at eye level and have small, appealing openings for curious fingers, resulting in countless electrocution-related injuries and even deaths each year. Plastic outlet covers and plugs are advised for injury avoidance, and childproof receptacles should preferable be used in place of normal outlets.

If you have upper-story windows, install childproof safety bars that are simple for adults to open in the event of a fire or other emergency. When children are present, keep windows closed and always secured, and never leave small children alone near open windows. Never expect a screen to keep a youngster from slipping out of a window. Keep items away from windows to avoid children from climbing on the sills. Most houses include a range of things, such as furniture, that may be pushed or climbed on, causing injury or death. Anti-tip devices are offered for dressers, bookshelves, entertainment centers, televisions, appliances, and tall floor lamps. Appliance locks are inexpensive, easy to install, and keep refrigerators and stoves securely closed to keep your child safe.

CAUTION!

The American Academy of Pediatrics does not endorse mobile baby walkers because they result in thousands of newborn head injuries each year. These hazardous, wheel-driven baby walkers are less prevalent anymore, and most professionals strongly advise against using them, so politely decline one, even if it's a hand-me-down.

Make sure the crib you choose meets federal safety regulations and keep the mattress in excellent shape. To avoid sudden infant death syndrome, never place a baby face down on a plastic-covered mattress or table (SIDS). Always elevate the side rails of your crib and fasten up children in safety-belted highchairs, strollers, and changing tables, among other things. To prevent falls, never leave your newborn alone on a bed, sofa, or changing table; instead, pick them up if you need to answer the phone or retrieve anything.

When you have babies and toddlers in the home, all your coffee tables, furniture, and worktops with sharp edges should have safety padding OR other professionally constructed coverings connected to the corners. Install hardware-mounted safety gates between any things you want to protect and at the top of each stairwell. Avoid using accordion gates, which may entrap a child's head, and pressure-mounted gates, which are inadequately secure.

NOTE!

Children under the age of eight should never be given balloons. Keep a watch on children of all ages while around balloons since they may quickly rupture, and minute parts can clog the airway if consumed. Since balloons cannot be seen on X-rays, it may be unclear why a child is uncomfortable if they have ingested a balloon piece.

Thin plastics provide a suffocation danger around babies and children and should be discarded immediately. Keep all plastic garbage bags and other plastic bags, such as sandwich bags, away from children. To prevent choking and strangling, take the following precautions:

- Nuts of any type, hard sweets, fruit with seeds, grapes, raw carrots, raw peas, raw celery, cherries with pits, or popcorn should not be given to children under the age of three.
- Avoid providing little children and babies clothes with drawstrings; remove drawstrings from waistbands, jackets, and hoods; and cut strings off mitts and other items (mobiles and crib toys).
- If your infant has outgrown just sleeping and looking at the mobile, take it down and secure it.
- Employ specially designed cable clamps or tie up window-blind cords out of reach.

- Use headbands and necklaces with care. On newborns, as well as anything that may possibly wrap around a baby's neck, such as hanging purses or diaper bags, lengthy telephone lines, and pacifiers secured around the neck.
- Never place your newborn face down on a soft surface such as a waterbed, sheepskin rug, quilt, mattress cover, soft cushion, beanbag, pillow loaded with beads, or next to a large stuffed animal.

> ***CAUTION!***
>
> *The thermostat on your home's hot water heater should be adjusted at 120°F or lower. If you live in an apartment and cannot control the water temperature, install an anti-scald device that causes the water to slow to a trickle if it reaches a dangerous level.*

Drowning is the greatest cause of mortality among children under the age of five. All pools and Jacuzzis need a pool fence with a self-closing, self-latching gate that prevents entrance to the water, pool alarms, and cautious adult supervision while children are present. Gadgets for children under the age of eight should never be used in lieu of parental supervision. After the youngsters have finished playing in a wading pool, drain the whole pool of water. Indeed, you should never leave any body of water alone, even buckets of water or other liquids since toddlers may drown in unattended buckets in minutes.

Never, ever leave a baby alone in a bath or wading pool, not even for a second to take a phone call. Pick up the baby and take him with you! Always stay in the bathroom when filling a tub with water.

Firearms should be stored in a locked case out of reach of youngsters. They must be manually unloaded and unlocked, and all drivers must have padlocks to prevent the cylinder from locking into place. Children should be educated and reminded that weapons are not toys and should never be acquired or used for recreational purposes.

Children and Toxic Threats

Every year, thousands of children enter emergency rooms because of accidental poisoning. Nowadays, safety latches and locks for cupboards and drawers designed to keep small hands out are available at any home improvement or general retail outlet.

According to EPA regulations, any homes built before 1978 that are being renovated should have their lead paint analyzed. Prior to 1978, any furniture, toys, or infant products could have been painted or finished with potentially hazardous levels of lead.

All pharmaceutical products, including over-the-counter medications and supplements, may pose a risk to one's health. Never try to trick your children into taking a vitamin or prescription by making it look like candy.

> ***NOTE!***
>
> *The main cause of poisoning-related death in children is accidental iron overdoses from children's vitamins. If you suspect your child has taken vitamins, store all your medicines in a safe place and notify the Poison Control Center immediately.*

Never sit on a counter while taking medications, including OTC medications, vitamins, and supplements. Even if a product is branded "kid resistant," it is not necessarily "childproof." Since 20% of accidental child poisonings occur when children are in the care of their grandparents, it is critical that grandparents and all other child caregivers be informed of the potential hazards of medications and vitamins, as well as the necessary safety steps.

Protecting the Elderly

Older persons often have less muscle mass and flexibility, and their bones may be porous and more brittle. Moreover, when their judgment and reaction times degrade, their senses of sight, hearing, touch, and smell are likely to suffer. Because of all these factors, the elderly is more vulnerable to accidents. The elderly must take precautions, including the following basic measures:

- Put emergency phone numbers next to each phone and have several cordless phones on hand if possible.

- Install door lever-action knobs that are easy to handle; keep door thresholds low and beveled; and avoid using throw rugs.
- Carpets and rugs should not be worn out, and nonskid backings should be used on loose rugs.
- Keep the railings and steps outside in excellent shape.
- Make use of both indoor and outdoor lights.
- Maintain a safe place for medications, ensure that all prescriptions are current, and discard any that have past their expiration date.
- Use either strips or a nonskid mat. Put grab bars on the walls next to the bathtub and toilet, as well as safety glass or plastic over the bathtub's standing area.

VITAL!

By keeping track of your prescriptions, you may avoid complications such as overdosing, mixing the wrong meds, taking excessive doses of the same kind of medication, and taking the incorrect medication. Create a note of the medication's name, intended use, dose instructions, pill color and shape, suggested times to take it, any safety warnings, the prescription date, and the pharmacy that is providing it.

Keep it Clean!

Dust, grime, and dust mites all contribute to sickness and allergies, and household clutter may lead to accidents. National Institute of Nursing Research found that homes who wash their garments in hot water and bleach had a 25% lower infection risk than households that DO NOT use bleach.

> ***VITAL!***
>
> *For cleaning and disinfecting, mix 1/4 cup household bleach with 1 gallon of room temperature water. Surfaces should be lightly misted with the mixture, then rinsed after 10 minutes.*

To help keep yourself and your house healthy and safe, follow these steps:

- Take out the trash every day.
- Wash your sheets at least once a week and all your bed linens once a week in hot water to avoid the creation of dust mites, which lead to allergies.
- Vacuuming your house on a regular basis will help keep allergies and dust at bay.
- Seal any cracks and gaps in the floor, as well as those near baseboards, fireplaces, and pipes, to keep dirt and insects out.

- Bathe pets once a month and keep them away from sofas, chairs, and beds to protect their fur and dander from infecting the house.

Note that antibacterial hand soaps kill both good and harmful germs, so use appropriate hand-washing techniques with mild soap and warm water instead of these products, even though they seem to be excellent sanitation goods.

Chapter 4

Typical In-Home Incidents

On any given day, injuries and accidents in the home are common among all families. People get harmed in ordinary activities, and diseases occur during life, which may range from moderate to severe. Some are treatable at home, while others need medical intervention.

Cuts (Lacerations)

Every day, cuts and abrasions of many types might occur, ranging from scraped knees to broken bones. To serious wounds on fingers and hands in the kitchen and workshop on a patio. Cuts are skin wounds that include skin separation and are often caused by a sharp instrument such as a knife or a piece of glass.

Follow the instructions below to care for minor cuts and abrasions:

1. Your hands should be washed with soap and water, and the wound should be washed under running water. Apply direct pressure with a sterile cloth or bandage to bleeding wounds and elevate the wound.
2. Use antibiotic cream, but avoid using iodine or hydrogen-peroxide solutions, which may cause more harm to wounded tissues and may trigger allergic responses in those who are sensitive to iodine and shellfish.

3. Treat the wound with a sterile gauze bandage, preferably nonstick, to protect it from infection and water loss until a scab forms.
4. Keep the wound area clean and replace any soiled dressings as soon as possible.

> ***CAUTION!***
>
> *Never clean a wound that is plainly infected. If you can't get it clean, carefully cover it in a sterile bandage and take it to the doctor.*

Change most dressings daily and change dressings when any fluids soak through, to reduce the possibility of the wound drying and sticking to the dressing. Cleaning up Open wounds may sometimes bleed, which may be quickly stopped with direct pressure applied with a sterile gauze pad.

First Aid for Deeper Cuts

In the instance of deep enough lacerations to reveal fatty tissue:

1. Bring the edges of the wound together and fix them with butter-fly closures.
2. Use an antiseptic OR antibacterial ointment. Over butterfly closures, bandage and seek medical treatment.

VITAL!

Never wash severe wounds since doing so may cause them to bleed faster. Removing blood-stained clothing from serious injuries may cause the bleeding to resume. Instead, place fresh dressings on top of the previous treatments until the bleeding stops.

Go see a doctor:

- For cuts that continue to bleed after 10 minutes or applying pressure
- If there is a possibility that nerves or tendons have been damaged.
- If anything is lodged in the cut
- If the cut was made by an animal or human bite, or if it was pierced by something unclean, infection is possible.
- Whether the cut is on the mouth, face, hand, or genitals, it is called a mouth cut.

If stitches are required, keep the wound closed with butterfly closures until you can see a doctor. If the wound is unclean OR is likely to be so, such as with human or animal attacks, you only have around six hours before it is too contaminated to stitch. Some wounds may goo as long as eight hours after the accident before being stitched, but the longer you wait, the less probable stitches will be feasible, and any scarring will be reduced.

Get urgent medical assistance if you notice any indicators of complications such as numbness OR reduced movement; discomfort, inflammation, swelling, or red streaks around the wound or fever.

> ***NOTE!***
>
> *If a cut is longer than one-half inch, is gaping open, and has edges that DO NOT stay together, contact your healthcare provider immediately since stitches are often necessary.*

Stop the Bleeding

As a wound begins to bleed, apply pressure to control the bleeding. Treat the wound as an emergency if it is deep and bleeding profusely. Control the bleeding by applying consistent direct pressure to the injury with a sterile gauze or pad. To assist avoid shock, lie the person down with their feet raised. Never apply direct pressure to a wound with a protruding Item OR bone; instead, apply pressure to both sides of the wound. If possible, raise the cut above the level of the person's heart, and if the bleeding is copious and continuous, refer to Chapter 2, Managing Shock, and contact 911 right away.

First Aid for Abrasions

While treating abrasions, follow these steps:

1. Remove any debris from an abrasion, such as dirt, fiber, and stones, before cleaning it.

2. Tweezers may be used to remove any little items. Wipe the wound gently in one direction using a non-occlusive wipe.
3. Wash wound with soap and water, apply antibiotic cream, and cover with a clean dressing.

Wounds from Puncture

A puncture wound is a small but deep hole caused by anything that can penetrate the skin deeply, such as fangs, needles, spears, staples, nails, or any other instrument. Puncture wounds seldom bleed much, but they may cause internal damage and it can be difficult to detect how deep the cut is.

First Aid for Puncture Wounds

Puncture wounds should always be considered unclean. To treat small wounds:

1. Wash your hands with soap and water and wear gloves.
2. As the wound is immersed in a stream of running water, clean it with soap and then with povidone-iodine.
3. Bandage loosely and check the area every day for infection-related signs such as edema, redness, or worsening discharge.

Avoid using antibiotic ointments and never seal puncture wounds to reduce the risk of infection. Avoid trying to clean a large puncture wound since this might result in more serious bleeding. Never try to extract a stuck object from a perforated wound. Depending on where the wound is placed, this might result in more harm, bleeding, or even death. Never attempt to press body fragments back into a wound, breathe on a wound, or probe for debris since doing so may result in a serious infection later.

Call 911 immediately if you have any significant puncture wounds. If the wound is bleeding heavily, apply direct pressure on it until help arrives.

QUESTION?

When should a bandage be changed?

Although there are no formal requirements for dressing changes, it is typically suggested to change bandages every day or anytime they get dirty or wet due to activity, blood, or other wound secretions.

Infections Caused by Cuts

Every time the skin is damaged, there is a risk of infection because cuts enable bacteria, viruses, and fungus to enter the body and cause diseases. Infections may develop locally (in a single place of the body) or spread throughout the body through the circulation (systemic infection). Warm or heated skin, localized soreness, pus-like discharge, redness and swelling, as well as a fever and chills, are all symptoms of a localized infection. Most localized, minor diseases may be treated at home using the following methods:

1. Every day, wash the area with soap and water.

2. Apply antibiotic cream or ointment to the affected region, then gently cover it in dry gauze with a nonstick bandage.
3. Watch for signs of a more serious infection, such as swelling, pain, increased redness, or pus.

A localized infection may evolve into a dangerous local infection known as cellulitis when the skin around the incision becomes raised, red, painful, and thicker in texture, along with symptoms such as enlarged lymph nodes, red streaks on the skin, fever, chills, and shaking. A local infection may spread throughout the body and cause symptoms such as fever, shaking, chills, widespread weakness, and joint pain. Consult your doctor if you have a localized infection that does not clear up in three days, if you have cellulitis or systemic infection symptoms, if you have infections of the face, particularly those near the eyes, if you are young or elderly, or if you or someone you know has an underlying medical condition. To prevent infection, wash your hands often, avoid picking or scratching sores or blemishes, wipe any cuts and scratches with soap and water, and keep wounds clean and bandaged.

Tooth Loss, Dental Pain, and Dental Injuries

Accidental tooth loss occurs more often than you may imagine, so you should consider include a tooth-preservation kit in your first-aid supplies. These kits are widely available at most pharmacies. The sooner you see a dentist for cavities or conditions that cause toothaches, the better.

How to Manage Accidental Tooth Loss

A knocked-out or partially dislodged tooth is often replaced in its socket within 30 minutes after an occurrence. Adults should use clean gauze to keep the tooth in place without contacting the root. If the tooth has gotten dirty, you may handle it with a sterile gauze or pad and rinse it with water, but cleaning a dislodged tooth is not recommended. If you are unable to keep the tooth in place for any reason, or if you cannot get to a dentist or emergency room within thirty minutes, the tooth may be placed in a jar with fresh whole milk or the individual's own saliva for transfer. To stop the bleeding, place a piece of sterile gauze or a pad over the cut and bite down. Maintain this pressure for twenty minutes, or until bleeding protocols are carried out.

> ***CAUTION!***
>
> *If a child's tooth came out due to an accident or injury, DO NOT try to replace it. A child's tooth may not be properly retained, or they may accidentally swallow it. Put the tooth in whole milk to keep it alive until a dentist can re-insert it (not powdered or skimmed).*

Broken Teeth

After cleaning the mouth with water, apply clean gauze over the shattered tooth. Apply a cold compress to the face to relieve pain and swelling. Save the shattered piece and contact your dentist; they may be able to reattach it. Before getting dental treatment, DO NOT eat or drink anything.

First Aid for Toothache

If your teeth become painfully sensitive to cold or heat, this could be a sign of gum disease or a problem with the nerve within the tooth. Daily use of sensitive tooth toothpaste may be used to treat sensitive teeth, but a trip to the dentist is required if you have a toothache.

- Astringent mouthwashes are antiseptic and help to reduce swelling in the early stages of toothache.
- Apply a cold pack to the face and take aspirin, ibuprofen, or acetaminophen for pain and swelling. (Remember, never give aspirin to children under the age of sixteen due to the risk of Reye's syndrome, a potentially deadly illness.)
- Wrap ice around your hands. According to Canadian research, rubbing an ice cube between your hands may ease dental pain because the icy, rubbing sensation follows the same brain route as tooth pain and generally overcomes signals from your mouth. Wrap a cube around the convergent bones of your thumb and index finger and stroke it.
- If the discomfort persists, see a dentist. A life-threatening abscessed tooth that is spreading from your tooth to other regions of your face requires quick medical or dental intervention.

Diabetic Emergencies

Diabetes impairs a person's capacity to generate and use insulin, which the body requires to convert sugar, starches, and other carbohydrates into energy. Diabetics who have high blood sugar levels for an extended period may go into a diabetic coma or lose consciousness.

What to Watch Out For

The following symptoms, as well as those associated with low or high blood sugar, may suggest the development of a diabetic coma:

- Deep and rapid breathing
- Fast heart rate
- Frequent urination
- Fruit-smelling breath
- Drowsiness
- Warm, dry, red skin
- Dry mouth
- Extreme thirst
- Agitation, change in behavior, irritation.
- Loss of consciousness
- Vomiting and Nausea with upper abdominal pain

NOTE!

A diabetic coma, a potentially lethal disease, may occur because of both hyperglycemia (very high blood sugar) and hypoglycemia (extremely low blood sugar).

Actions to Take

If you have hyperglycemia or hypoglycemia, you should do the following:

1. If you know a person has diabetes or locate a medical alert bracelet that says she has diabetes, ask her whether she has taken her prescribed insulin. If she hasn't, or you're unsure, call 911.
2. If she suffers hypoglycemia, give her some sugar, such as fruit juice. Avoid feeding hard candy to persons who are seriously ill or in a weakened state due to the risk of choking.

Many individuals are aware of how to check their blood glucose levels and manage their diabetes. If the measured blood sugar remains below 60 mg/dL or the individual continues to display signs of severe hypoglycemia, hyperglycemia, or an insulin response, call 911 and proceed to the nearest emergency facility.

> ***VITAL!***
>
> *Try using "The Bottle of Life," a huge prescription bottle embossed on the top and sides with enormous red crosses, as an EMS notification method. First responders are instructed to look for a piece of paper with a list of all medications and medical conditions that is kept inside the refrigerator with the bottle.*

Earache and Ear Injury

The most frequent causes of earaches are otitis media, an infection of the middle ear, and otitis externa, sometimes known as swimmer's ear, an inflammation of the outer ear canal. Some of the reasons include minor ear canal injury, fluid accumulation in the inner ear, or germs, which leads in discomfort, swelling, and pain. Earaches are not communicable; they mostly affect older children and are occasionally associated with bottle feeding, pacifier use, second-hand smoking, and allergies.

An earache may cause severe stabbing pain, loss of hearing, itching, fever, nausea, or vomiting. Additional symptoms include ear enlargement, ringing or buzzing sounds, and fluids draining from the ear.

First Aid for Earache

If you have a fever or an ear discharge, get medical attention immediately once; if an infection is the cause of your earache, treatment will be necessary. Do the following steps:

- Children should be examined on a regular basis by a doctor.
- Antibiotics should be administered till the end.
- To relieve discomfort, use eardrops, heating packs, and over-the-counter drugs such ibuprofen, acetaminophen, and aspirin (only for adults).
- Wash hands often to help avoid ear infections.

- A bulb syringe may be used to gently suction mucus out of an infant's or toddler's nose. During feeding, keep the baby's head up.
- Raise the head of a child's bed a few inches (place item under the mattress, not on top where it may lead to suffocation) to help drain the fluid that collects behind the eardrums and use a humidifier in your child's room at night.

Never put matches, hairpins, cotton-tipped swabs, or anything else in your ear. This may cause substantial ear damage by pushing wax further into the ear canal or perforating the eardrum.

How to Treat an Ear Injury

Ear injuries are often linked with pain, dizziness, loss of hearing, and internal bleeding. Take these steps to treat an ear injury:

1. DO NOT attempt to seal the ear or stop any bleeding; instead, wrap the exterior of the ear loosely with a bandage or dressing to absorb any blood and drainage.
2. Lay the individual on their injured side with the damaged ear facing down to drain the blood. Then, call 911 or go to an emergency room right away.

Food Poisoning

Any activity involving food might result in food poisoning or food-borne illness. Clean your hands before commencing any cooking or cleaning in the kitchen and use separate cutting boards for each operation to avoid cross-contamination. Always wash fresh produce before chopping, cutting, or eating it. While handling meat, follow the directions on the package labels. If you have any worries about the freshness of any food in your refrigerator, discard it.

There are two forms of food poisoning: infectious agents and poisonous agents. The most prevalent infectious agents are viruses, bacteria, and parasites. Poisonous agents include pesticides on fruits and vegetables, deadly mushrooms, and poorly prepared foreign cuisine. When a specific contamination is detected, viruses and bacteria are usually to blame. Poisonous agents are generally the consequence of the creation of dangerous food or other rare instances, such as gathering wild mushrooms, and therefore DO NOT cause food poisoning as often as infectious agents.

Pesticides, such as those found on unwashed vegetables or fruits, may cause mild to severe sickness, with symptoms such as shaking arms and legs, heightened sensitivity, impaired vision, headaches, cramps, and diarrhea. Manufacturers have lately had to recall various items due to contamination, which has resulted in illness and even death.

First Aid for Food Poisoning

In treating food poisoning, use the following advice:

- Avoiding solid meals during the nausea and vomiting phase and drinking enough of fluids, especially clear liquids, are the best methods to care for someone at home who has short bouts of vomiting and little quantities of diarrhea that last less than twenty hours.

- Avoid alcoholic, caffeinated, and sugary beverages in favor of over-the-counter rehydration solutions designed specifically for children, such as Pedialyte and Rehydralyte, as well as diluted sports drinks such as Gatorade and Powerade (full-strength energy drinks contain too much sugar and may cause diarrhea in adults).
- After the nausea and vomiting have eased and you can tolerate fluids, gradually resume normal food intake with easy-to-digest items such as rice, wheat cereals and bread, potatoes, bland cereals, lean meats, and baked chicken. Milk is safe to drink unless you have lactose sensitivity.

Most of the time, OTC drugs are not required to treat diarrhea, while they are frequently safe when taken as directed and only by adults. If you have any worries or symptoms of dehydration, such as nausea, vomiting, or diarrhea that lasts more than 24 hours, bloody diarrhea, and/or a high fever, get medical attention.

Allergic Reactions

An allergic reaction is an acquired, abnormal inflammatory response to an allergen that is mild to moderate in most individuals. Pollens, medications, certain foods, insect stings and bites, dust mites, pet dander, scents, and detergents may all trigger an allergic reaction. Allergies affect people of all ages, and reactions to allergens may range from mild to severe, including anaphylaxis, a potentially deadly allergic reaction. Even though a person may have previously had no or only very moderate reactions to an allergen for many years, repeated exposures (sensitization) may eventually result in a more severe reaction without warning in some conditions. Even little exposure to an allergen might result in a potentially catastrophic reaction as you grow increasingly sensitive to it.

CAUTION!

Anybody with a history of severe allergies should carry an epinephrine auto-injector pen with written instructions on how and when to use it, as well as a Medical Alert ID or tag. A doctor's prescription is required for the self-care epinephrine injector, and a medic alert bracelet may be obtained by dialing 1-800-ID- ALERT.

Allergies occur when the immune system, the body's defensive mechanism, meets anything it considers as a foreign object and a risk through eating, touching, breathing, or injecting. In certain circumstances, your immune system can protect your body, but it might be difficult to distinguish between serious risks and innocuous substances. These extremely sensitive systems often have an inflammatory response to items such as certain meals that aren't harmful. Allergies may range from mild to severe, requiring immediate medical attention. Symptoms may be localized and present straight away, or they can be widespread (systemic) and develop over time.

Warning Signs and Symptoms

Even though most allergic reactions are mild, it is always a good idea to notify your doctor if the disease is new or unrelated to your medical history. Moderate allergic reactions may result in the following symptoms:

- Itchy, runny nose with clear nasal discharge
- Itchy, watery eyes
- Itchy skin
- Minor swelling
- Rashes and hives
- Sneezing

Mild Reactions

Preventing contact with the allergen may help prevent an itchy, localized rash (contact dermatitis). Keep the area clean and dry, wash away any known allergies with soap and water straight soon, and treat with calamine lotion if required. See your family doctor to determine if antihistamines, decongestant medicines, or a combination of the two are appropriate for all allergy symptoms. To treat rashes, your doctor may suggest you use antihistamine cream or cream containing 1% hydrocortisone. The best line of action is to identify and prevent whatever is causing the allergic reaction.

Sinus Irrigation for Mild Allergies

Sinus irrigation is a procedure for flushing and irrigating the sinuses and the inside of the nose to alleviate allergies. It also helps with breathing by cleaning out any infection that may be forming in your nasal passages and aggravating your sinuses. To prevent nasal tissue swelling and tissue injury, an isotonic salt solution (salt concentration equivalent to that of your body) must be used. You may buy commercial items. To make your own solution, combine 1-pint warm water, 1/2 teaspoon salt, and 1/2 teaspoon baking soda. Keep it in the fridge for up to 2 weeks.

To reduce nasal congestion caused by allergies, use the sinus irrigation approach outlined below:

1. Use a soft rubber-tip bulb syringe to irrigate the nose.
2. Hold your head forward, your mouth open, and your chin out over a sink or in the shower.
3. Pause breathing and insert the tip of the bulb syringe into your nose. Squeeze the fluid into your nostrils, taking care not to swallow. If you need to swallow, pause, lean forward, and let the solution pour out of your nose.
4. Repeat on the opposite side, and then blow your nose lightly while shutting your lips on each side.

If you are bothered by airborne allergens, clean your sinuses twice a day at first, then every day to every third day OR after allergen-exposure-related activities. You may also use a pulsating system if the manufacturer's instructions are followed.

> ***NOTE!***
>
> *Never assume you are entirely protected just because you or a family member receives allergy shots. Families with known allergies should be especially aware about CPR and the use of epinephrine auto-injectors in emergency circumstances.*

Severe Allergic Reactions

Severe allergic reactions, which occur less often, may be deadly if not treated promptly. If someone exhibits any of the following symptoms, take them to a hospital emergency department straight once, or call 911 for emergency transportation right away:

- Signs of panic or anxiety
- Rapid breathing
- Swelling of the face, eyes, tongue, or lips.
- Flushed face, neck, chest, arms, hands, feet, or tongue.
- Dizziness or weakness
- Nausea and / or vomiting.
- Abdominal cramping or pain
- A feeling of tightness in the chest and throat
- Feeling faint or loss of consciousness
- Lips turning blue.
- Difficulty swallowing
- Difficulty breathing and wheezing.
- Pale and damp skin

After a severe allergic response, the brain and other vital organs may lose oxygen owing to airway swelling. If someone is experiencing these symptoms, it is critical that they get prompt help; therefore, call 911 and follow the emergency response procedures outlined in Chapter 2.

Anaphylactic Shock

If quick treatment is not given, a person may die from anaphylaxis, a severe systemic (whole-body) allergic reaction, in less than 15 minutes. Anaphylaxis is characterized by the following symptoms:

- Heart palpitations (missed beats)
- Weak or rapid pulse
- Abnormal breathing sounds
- Confusion
- Wheezing
- Difficulty breathing
- Hives
- Dizziness
- Lightheadedness
- Fainting
- Slurred speech
- Skin turning blue (including the lips and nail beds)
- Cough
- Nasal congestion
- Diarrhea

- Nausea and vomiting
- Anxiety
- Itching and redness of skin

> ***CAUTION!***
>
> *Doctors will prescribe an epinephrine auto-injector to patients with severe allergies. If someone in your family who has a prescription is suffering a severe allergic response indicated by a constriction of the neck and trouble breathing, you must use the injector immediately as advised by their doctor.*

Without early treatment, these symptoms, which commonly emerge in seconds or minutes in response to an allergen, may result in anaphylactic shock, which can include dangerously low blood pressure, respiratory arrest (the individual stops breathing), and cardiac arrest (when the heart stops beating).

Keep your cool. To avoid significant allergic reactions, follow the steps below:

1. Call 911 straight away.
2. Check the for ABCs (airway, breathing, and circulation). Details on CPR method may be found in Chapter 2.
3. If a person has been stung by a bee, they should use a knife, credit card, or fingernail to remove the stinger without touching the attached bag (see Chapter 5). If possible, keep the sting site below the level of the person's heart while

washing the area with soap and water and applying a cold pack.

4. If the individual can breathe easily, lie them down with their head tilted up (DO NOT use a pillow as this might obstruct breathing) and elevate their feet by eight to twelve inches to prevent shock. A blanket may be used to keep the individual warm. If the individual is having trouble breathing, place them in a sitting position and keep them quiet until EMS comes.
5. DO NOT provide the individual food or drink if they are wheezing, having problems breathing, or swallowing.

Chapter 5

Outdoor Incidents

In a variety of seasons and climates, the great outdoors is an excellent place to work, play, travel, and entertain. Critters that live outdoors (or are supposed to) may annoy or damage humans, and heat and cold can also be harmful. You may also feel ill if you don't drink enough water or if you have other severe ailments. Whatever you do outdoors, it is important to understand how to care for and assist people who may get injuries or illnesses because of your actions.

Bites from Insects, Animals, and Humans

A variety of insects and animals, including humans, may bite or sting you, resulting in painful or lethal bites and stings ranging in intensity from mild to moderate to severe. It is critical to understand how to react, address, and seek care for any of these potential injuries.

Bites from Scorpions

Scorpions are lobster-like arachnid arthropods (the same class as spiders) that are commonly found in dry parts of the Southwest and Mexico. They have a stinger that curls at the end of their tail. Although scorpion stings are unlikely to be fatal and are easily treated, children and the elderly are more vulnerable than adults.

Some of the symptoms include immediate pain or burning, mild swelling, sensitivity to touch, and a numb or tingling sensation.

The following steps should be taken for scorpion bite treatment:

1. Clean the area using soap and water.
2. Apply a cold pack to the affected area for ten minutes, repeat as needed at ten-minute intervals.
3. Contact the Poison Control Center if you have any severe symptoms.

Bites from Ticks

People who live near forested and grassy areas, or who frequent these areas for recreation, are more likely to suffer tick bites. Since they feed on the blood of mammals such as deer, rats, and rabbits, these little spiders may transfer disease from animals to people.

To reduce the chance of getting a tick-borne infectious illness such as Lyme disease, Colorado tick fever, or Rocky Mountain spotted fever, the first aid for tick bites is to remove the tick as quickly as possible.

To get rick of a tick:

1. Using a pair of flat or curved forceps tweezers, carefully remove the tick's head as near to the skin as possible without crushing the tick.
2. After cleaning the affected area with soap and water, use 1% hydrocortisone antihistamine lotion.

Get medical attention. If the tick is too deeply embedded to be removed, you live in an area where Lyme disease is a risk, you develop a fever and flu-like symptoms, muscle weakness or paralysis, or the bull's-eye rash that is a symptom of Lyme disease, you may be at risk.

CAUTION!

Ticks will dig deeper if petroleum jelly, alcohol, or ammonia are applied to them. If you reside in a high-risk area and suffer a tick bite, always seek medical advice since you may need further medical care, such as antibiotics.

Bites from Animals

Cats and dogs are the most often bitten animals. Cat bites can result in extremely deep puncture wounds and pose a significant risk of infection because punctures force germs deep into the skin and tissues. Dog bites can increase the chance of infection and tissue damage. These bites frequently result in markings where the skin has split and sometimes bleeding, depending on the degree and location of the bites. Redness and swelling usually appear between twenty-four and forty-eight hours.

VITAL!

Raccoons, stray dogs, rats, and bats are examples of wild animals that may enter your home and pose a much larger risk since they are more likely to carry and spread illnesses such as rabies and other viruses. These types of bites should be treated by a doctor as soon as possible.

Consult a veterinarian about potential health risks following an animal bite, and have the wounds examined by a doctor. Your doctor may advise you to get a tetanus shot and, in some cases, antibiotics. Keep the pet safe and secure in your home until a doctor examines the bite and the appropriate health authorities rule out any communicable diseases.

Assess the sufferer's airway, breathing, and circulation, and begin CPR (see Chapter 2) if the bite is severe or the person loses consciousness. Following then, call 911 and treat the shock until help arrives. Follow the steps below for minor bites:

1. After thoroughly cleaning your hands with soap and water, wash the bite in running water for at least five minutes.
2. To clean the bite, use soap, water, saline solution, and or povidone-iodine.
3. For cuts and lacerations, treat the bite as instructed, then apply direct pressure to stop the bleeding.
4. Put a cold pack on undamaged skin.
5. Elevate the wounded limb above the level of the person's heart, if possible, to reduce swelling.
6. Every day, keep a watch out for infection signs like as swelling, redness, or discharge at the bite site.

Large and deep puncture wounds need medical attention. Since bites to your hands, neck, or face may cause serious sickness and/or scarring, you should always seek medical assistance.

> ***CAUTION!***
>
> *Instead of trying to catch a wild animal, contact animal control and the police. If it's a pet, contact the owner and inquire whether it's been vaccinated against rabies. In situations of animal bites, the animal must be checked for rabies and reported to authorities.*

Bites from Humans

Human bites are possibly more dangerous than animal bites due to the enormous number of germs and viruses prevalent in human lips. Human bites provide a substantial risk of infection. Infections, such as joint infections, may have devastating implications, even in minor wounds. Avoid putting a human bite wound in your mouth since this will introduce germs to the wound. For human bites, take the following precautions:

1. If the skin around the wound is not injured, thoroughly clean it with soap and water or saline. Never attempt to clean the wound from a human bite that is actively bleeding.
2. Apply antibiotic cream to the wound, cover it with a nonstick bandage, and monitor the area closely.
3. Get medical attention if there is numbness or if the fingers cannot be bent or straightened.
4. If the skin is injured and bleeding, apply direct pressure with a clean, dry towel to stop the bleeding. Elevate the area,

cover the wound with a sterile bandage, and seek medical attention.

5. To minimize problems from any severe wounds, get medical attention as soon as possible after being bitten.

If you experience any infection signs, such as swelling, soreness, pus discharge, or tendon or nerve injury symptoms, such as trouble bending or straightening your finger or a loss of feeling over the tip of your finger, get medical attention.

Bites from Spiders

Only the bites of two spiders known in the United States, the brown recluse and black widow, are potentially lethal to humans. Some tarantula species may cause severe but non-life-threatening local reactions. Understanding what sort of spider bit, you may regularly aid in treatment and may even save your life.

Numbness at the bite site, disorientation, sweating, skin rash, strong muscular and chest pain and muscle spasms, severe stomach cramps, nausea and vomiting, trouble breathing, and chest tightness are all signs of a black-widow spider bite. These symptoms might emerge anywhere between one and twenty-four hours following the bite. White blisters that may occasionally grow into painful ulcers (craters), a rash, swelling, and stiffness, weakness, backache, joint pain, and fever are all potential symptoms.

> ***VITAL!***
>
> *The appropriate treatment will be determined by the kind of spider; thus, if you can kill or catch the spider without placing yourself in danger, do so and bring it with you to the emergency department. Nevertheless, there is no antivenom available for tarantula or brown recluse bites.*

First Aid Treatment for Spider Bites

The following steps should be performed in the event of a spider bite:

1. If you feel you were bitten by a nonpoisonous spider, wash the bite site, treat it as indicated for cuts and lacerations, cover the bite with a clean bandage, and see a doctor if any infection signs arise.
2. For any black widow or brown recluse spider bites, call 911 or go to an emergency hospital straight soon to get treatment and, in the case of black widow bites, receive antivenom.
3. Observe the person's ABCs (see Chapter 2) and place them in a sitting position.

Bites from Snakes

Rattlesnakes, copperheads, cottonmouths (water moccasins), oral snakes, and cobras are among the numerous venomous snakes. Among the symptoms of a snake bite are:

- Diarrhea
- Seizures
- Warmth and burning at the sight of the bite.
- Blurred vision.
- Bleeding
- Loss of muscle coordination
- Increased thirst
- Fever
- Fainting
- Sweating
- Dizziness
- Skin discoloration and swelling
- Severe pain at the site of the bite
- Rapid heart rate
- Numbness and tingling
- Nausea and vomiting
- Weakness
- Fangs marks in the skin

A nonpoisonous snakebite will often leave a horseshoe-shaped ring of teeth marks on the victim's skin, producing little pain and edema.

First Aid Treatment for Snake Bites

The following are some non-poisonous snake bites first aid procedures:

1. Cleaning the bite with soap and water

2. Using sterile bandage or dressing to cover the affected area.

If you're unsure when your last tetanus vaccination was, see your doctor or inquire about a booster injection.

Bite swelling and color changes are common indicators of a venomous snake bite. To avoid a painful snakebite, follow these steps:

1. Call 911 and the Poison Control Center as soon as possible so that antivenom is available when the individual arrives at the emergency department.
2. To reduce venom circulation, relax the individual, limit movement, and keep the affected area below heart level.
3. Remove any jewelry or other constraining things from the region and use a light splint to help limit mobility.
4. If possible, keep track of your body's temperature, pulse, breathing rate, and blood pressure. Managing signs of shock indicated in Chapter 2.

Note that snakes may bite for up to an hour after they die, and DO NOT bring the dead snake inside until it is safe to do so. Don't make the person who has been bitten strain; if you need to move him, carry him. DO NOT use cold compresses or a tourniquet on the bite. Never try to suction or cut the poison out of a bite. DO NOT give the individual any medications or food or water until ordered to do so by a doctor.

Stings from Insects

Most individuals have modest responses to entity stings. Nonetheless, many stings, stings to the mouth and throat, and stings to those who have had a negative reaction to the venom must be treated as soon as possible, as described in Chapter 4.

First Aid Treatment for Insect Stings

First aid procedure for stings includes:

1. Wash the sting area using soap and water.
2. If necessary, use an ice pack to minimize swelling.
3. If possible, keep the sting area below the person's heart.

Calamine lotion and Benadryl (diphenhydramine hydrochloride) may also be used to relieve swelling and irritation. A combination of baking soda and water, together with uncoated aspirin, may also help to relieve stinging and inflammation.

If a person has been stung by a bee, they should:

1. Scrape the stinger away with a knife, credit card, or fingernail, without touching the attached sack. The sack will continue to inject venom into the wound.
2. Using tweezers or compressing the sack may result in the injection of more venom into the victim.
3. After cleansing the area with soap and water, apply an ice pack, if possible, keeping the sting site below the level of the person's heart.

Keep an eye out for signs of an allergic reaction, which may emerge up to twenty hours after being stung by a bee. If the website gets contaminated, see a doctor.

In the case of an allergic reaction, anaphylactic shock, or repeated stings, dial 911 or proceed to the nearest emergency facility for treatment and monitoring. Repeated stings in otherwise healthy persons might result in potentially deadly reactions.

Poison Ivy, Oak, and Sumac

More than half of the individuals in the United States experience an itchy, burning rash after coming into touch with poison ivy, poison oak, or poison sumac. Poison ivy is a vine or a shrub that has smooth leaves with slightly notched edges and grows in clusters of three. It is possible to find it east of the Rockies Mountains. Poison oak is a little shrub with smooth-edged leaves that grow in groups of three, five, or seven. It is exclusively found west of the Rockies. Poison sumac grows in wet areas in the southeast and has smooth, oval-shaped leaves with seven to thirteen on per stalk. Each of these plants could have a varied appearance dependent on the region and the sea.

> ***NOTE!***
>
> *The rash may not appear if plant oils are removed within ten minutes. Any oils on your skin may be removed with rubbing alcohol or a thorough wash with soap and water.*

Symptoms of Poison Ivy, Oak, and Sumac Rash

When sensitive people are exposed to any of these plants, an itchy rash usually appears between twenty-four and seventy-two hours later. The earliest signs of the rash are little red pimples that grow into blisters of varying sizes. The rash may crust or ooze, and it is typically in streaks (straight lines), but it may take any shape or pattern, and it may seem to spread since different sections of the body may develop a rash at different times.

First Aid Treatment for Poison Ivy, Oak, and Sumac Rash

Although blisters may break, the fluid from them does not transmit the rash; rather, it is transferred via direct contact with any oil that may remain on hands, clothes, or shoes, as well as any other items that function as carriers. Lighting campfires in poison ivy-infested areas needs particular care since the smoke from a burning poison ivy plant may be lethal if ingested. If you encounter any of these plants or their oils:

1. Wash as quickly as possible with soap and water.
2. Cold compresses wet with water or milk, calamine lotion, an oatmeal bath, and oral antihistamines such as Benadryl (diphenhydramine hydrochloride) and 1% hydrocortisone may help ease symptoms.
3. If you're feeling dizzy, lie down with your legs up over your head to increase blood flow to your brain.

4. If you begin to wheeze or have difficulty breathing, try an inhaled bronchodilator such as albuterol or epinephrine to open the airway. If you have been given epinephrine, use it as advised.

In addition, your doctor may recommend oral steroids to treat your poison ivy.

Frostbite and Hypothermia

Cold injuries may occur because of continuous exposure to cold weather or sudden exposure to very cold temperatures. Frostbite is a sort of cold injury that affects the skin's outer layer, while hypothermia is a type of cold injury that affects the center of the body. Even though they often occur concurrently, each of them may be experienced individually. In response to a chilly environment, the body constricts blood vessels, decreasing blood flow to the extremities, especially the fingers and toes, and releases hormones that stimulate shivering to increase heat generating.

Frostbite

Frostbite occurs when tissues are exposed to temperatures below the freezing point of skin. Just the nose, cheeks, ears, fingers, and toes are affected by this illness. Frostbite may be minor or profound. The symptoms of superficial frostbite include burning, numbness, tingling, itching, and chilly feelings. Affected areas seem white and frozen, yet they still resist touch. Severe frostbite symptoms include a loss of sensation at first, followed by a total loss of feeling.

Other symptoms include swelling, blood-filled blisters, and white or yellowish skin that seems waxy and becomes purple blue when heated. When pressed, the area becomes tough and offers little resistance, sometimes seeming dead and darkened. Deep frostbite causes extreme agony that lasts for weeks to months as healthy tissue recovers and separates from dead tissue when blood flow is restored, and the area is warmed. A dull, continuous hurting and throbbing sensation follows the suffering.

First Aid Treatment for Frostbite

If you see any signs of frostbite, follow these steps:

1. If possible, leave the area and seek help while keeping the affected region elevated.
2. Remove any jewelry or other objects that may be impeding blood flow and begin hydrating with non-alcoholic, non-caffeinated drinks.
3. Use a dry, sterile dressing to treat frostbitten fingers or toes, separate the damaged regions with cotton, and then go to a medical institution as quickly as possible.
4. Never attempt to rewarm a frostbitten area since doing so may cause it to freeze again, and the freezing and thawing cycle is very hazardous.
5. Avoid rubbing the frozen area with anything, since this might aggravate the tissue (the amount of tissue damage is directly related to the time frozen, not to the degree of temperature).

Hypothermia

Hypothermia occurs when your body's temperature regulation mechanisms are unable to keep you at a normal temperature for an extended period when exposed to low temperatures or cold, damp environments. Shivering, slurred speech, sluggish breathing, chilly, pale skin, lack of coordination, tiredness, lethargy, and apathy may occur if your internal body temperature falls below 95 degrees Fahrenheit. Hypothermia is more common in children and the elderly.

First Aid Treatment for Hypothermia

For hypothermia first-aid, follow these steps:

1. As you wait for help, dial 911 and take care of the person's airway, breathing, and circulation as outlined in Chapter 2.
2. If possible, move the person away from the cold and, at the absolute least, try to shelter them from the wind and the old ground.
3. Taking off all the people's wet garments and covering them with a lovely, dry blanket. Never use direct heat with a hot water bottle or a heating pad; instead, apply warm packs to the neck, chest wall, and groin. Attempting to warm up the arms and legs will send cold blood back to the heart, lungs, and brain, resulting in a severe drop in core body temperature.
4. If the individual is not vomiting, give them warm, non-alcoholic beverages. When a person suffering from

hypothermia is at risk of cardiac arrest, touch them with caution and avoid stroking or caressing them.

Snow Blindness

Snow blindness occurs when the eyes are exposed to UV radiation from the sun's strongly reflected light on snow. Symptoms of snow blindness include:

- Gritty sensation in the eyes that worsens as the eyelids move.
- Watering of the eyes
- Redness of the eyes
- Headache
- Increased pain in the eyes on exposure to light

First Aid Treatment for Snow Blindness

To treat snow blindness, you should:

1. Blindfold the individual, give them some rest, and remind them not to expose themselves again.
2. If you can't get the individual out of the sunlight, use the darkest bandages or sunglasses you have, to protect their eyes.

Once out of the light, the eyes normally recover in a few days with no long-term consequences. If there is even a remote possibility of snow blindness, always wear sunglasses. Don't wait until the disco starts to put on your sunglasses.

Dehydration

When you're dehydrated, your body doesn't have as much water and fluids as it should. Dehydration may occur because of drinking too many liquids, not enough fluid, or both. Dehydration may be mild, moderate, or severe depending on how much fluid is lost or not restored in the body. Severe dehydration is a life-threatening condition. Vomiting, diarrhea, excessive urine, excessive sweating, and fever all cause fluid loss in the body. If you are dehydrated owing to nausea, lack of appetite while sick, or mouth or throat sores, you may not be obtaining enough fluids. Among the signs of dehydration are:

- Lack of tearing
- Urine appearing dark yellow.
- Decrease or no urine output.
- Dry or sticky mouth
- For babies, the soft spot on the top of their head (fontanelle) will be markedly sunken.
- Lethargy and coma (in severe dehydration)
- Sunken eyes

Children and the elderly are more likely to suffer from dehydration.

First Aid Treatment for Dehydration

Mild dehydration may be treated using the following methods:

1. Take little, regular sips of drink rather than a large one at once, which may cause you to vomit. Sugary sports drinks, which may aggravate diarrhea, should be avoided. Electrolyte solutions are very useful in this respect. Instead of using plain water to rehydrate toddlers and newborns, use commercial electrolyte solutions such as Pedialyte.
2. In addition to treating the underlying cause of the ailment, hospitalization and intravenous fluids are occasionally necessary to treat severe dehydration. For symptoms like:

- Dizziness
- Lightheadedness
- Lethargy
- Confusion
- Lack of tears

Infants less than two months old have diarrhea or vomiting, little to no urine production in an eight-hour period, sunken eyes, dry skin that sticks up like a tent when pressed, quick pulse, blood in the stool or vomit, or listlessness, and lethargy.

NOTE!

Don't wait till you're thirsty to consume fluids. Instead, stay hydrated since fluids take two hours to begin functioning on your body and you are already dehydrated by the time you feel thirsty.

Everyone should drink enough of fluids every day, but they should drink much more in hot weather and when exercising. When you're unwell, don't wait for indications of dehydration; instead, attempt to push fluids or seek medical treatment.

Heat Emergencies

Heat cramps, heat exhaustion, and heat stroke are the three severity levels of heat crises. Measures in hot temperatures may help prevent all three of these. The most prevalent causes of heat crises include high temperatures, humidity, dehydration, severe or excessive activity, overdressing in hot conditions, alcohol intake, prescription usage (especially diuretics and psychiatric medicines), cardiovascular illness, and sweat gland malfunction. Heat illness is more common in children, the elderly, and obese adults than in other demographic categories, yet anybody may acquire it by ignoring the signs.

Heat Illness Symptoms

Early warning symptoms of heat illness include:

- Fatigue
- Profuse sweating
- Muscle cramps
- Thirst

Later symptoms include:

- Headache

- Lightheadedness
- Dizziness
- Darkened urine
- Cool, moist skin
- Nausea and vomiting
- Weakness

As heat illness intensifies and progresses to heatstroke, the following symptoms appear:

- Dry, hot, and red skin
- Rapid, shallow breathing
- Extreme confusion
- Irrational behavior
- Temperature above 104° Fahrenheit
- Seizures
- Weak, rapid heart rate
- Loss of consciousness
- Coma
- Death

First Aid Treatment for Heat Illness

If there are any signs of shock, convulsions, or loss of consciousness, dial 911 immediately and then control the airway, breathing, and circulation as indicated in Chapter 2. In non-emergency cases of heat sickness, take the following steps:

1. Put the individual on their back, with their feet elevated about 12 inches.
2. To reduce body temperature, use a fan, cool, moist towels, and covered cold packs on the person's neck, groin, and armpits.
3. Give the person a half cup of fluids every fifteen minutes, ideally a drink made from a quart of cold water and a teaspoon of salt.
4. Massage stiff muscles gently yet firmly.

Take note of the following:

- Don't give out fever-reducing medications like aspirin or acetaminophen since they may be dangerous in situations of heat exhaustion.
- Never use rubbing alcohol.
- If the individual is vomiting or behaving strangely, give them nothing to eat or drink.
- Never provide salt pills or drinks containing alcohol or caffeine since they disrupt the body's internal temperature regulation system.

Never underestimate the severity of heat illness, particularly in small children, the elderly, or the injured. Get medical attention if any symptoms persist after therapy.

Stings from Jellyfish

Jellyfish are gelatinous saltwater animals that are elongated and bell-shaped. Its tentacles may grow to be more than three feet long. Jellyfish venom often produces allergic reactions, including redness, severe pain from stinging, and raised welts. After that, other symptoms such as nausea, vomiting, diarrhea, back and stomach pain, a fever, chills, and sweating, as well as lymph node enlargement, may emerge. When the reaction is severe, a person may have difficulty breathing, faint out, or even die.

First Aid Treatment for Jellyfish Stings

Anybody experiencing severe symptoms such as agonizing pain, chest discomfort, or shortness of breath should seek medical attention immediately. Call 911, take care of any warning signs, and begin CPR as stated in Chapter 2. Other answers should take the following steps:

1. Fresh water will aggravate the irritation, so rinse with saltwater instead. Avoid using cold packs or massaging the affected area. To remove eye stings, use one gallon of fresh water.
2. For stings, use one-fourth strength vinegar and 5% acetic acid (white vinegar) or isopropyl alcohol; never use vinegar if you have oral edema or difficulty swallowing.
3. Remove any tentacles with tweezers while wearing gloves.
4. Apply a baking soda, mud, or shaving cream paste to the wound before shaving it with a razor or knife and repeating

the vinegar or alcohol application. During shaving, the paste will prevent additional toxin release.

5. To prevent the spread of the toxin, restrict mobility in the affected area. (For box jellyfish stings, bandage the injured region until you can receive medical treatment, wrapping it like a sprained ankle and ensuring the fingers and toes are still pink.)
6. To relieve itching, use 1% hydrocortisone cream two to three times day, as directed, and take over-the-counter pain relievers or antihistamines such as Benadryl.

If you still experience redness and irritation after two to three days, your doctor may prescribe topical and oral steroids. This suggests that the injury may be bacterially contaminated, and you should consult a doctor. Keep in mind that allergic reactions to jellyfish stings may occur up to four weeks later, so keep a look out for any signs.

Chapter 6

Events Anywhere

Everyone has minor aches and pains in daily life. From a headache to stomach discomfort, prevention and treatment may offer you with comfort and aid while also preventing minor health issues from becoming more severe. Whether you sustain an unintentional injury, have a chronic condition like asthma, or exhibit a symptom like a fever, knowing and using the right preventive, management, and treatment strategies is the key to maintaining your health.

Burns (Thermal, Chemical, and Other)

Burn injuries are among the most frequent and painful. Very high temperatures (both dry and wet), chemicals, electricity, radiation, and even extremely low temperatures may all cause burns. They might affect the lungs, skin, eyes, and other internal organs. A burn's intensity is often classified into one of three categories based on the depth of the burn and the subsequent damage.

1. First-degree burns, also known as superficial burns, affect just the epidermis, or outermost layer of skin. When treated early and without the development of blisters, first-degree burns frequently recover nicely. Sunburns are a common kind of first-degree burns.

2. Second-degree burns are more serious because they affect a deeper layer of skin and are more prone to infection. Partial-thickness burns are another term for them. Second-degree burns are the most painful because more tissue is damaged, yet nerve endings remain. These burns heal rapidly and DO NOT need medical care unless they are more than two to three inches in diameter or involve the hands, face, buttocks, penis, or vaginal area.
3. The most serious burns are third-degree burns, sometimes known as full-thickness burns since they involve every layer of skin. Although third-degree burns may cause only little discomfort, the skin may appear white, black, or leathery, and the surrounding areas may be quite painful. All third-degree burns require medical attention. Call 911 for assistance and transportation or take the victim to the nearest emergency hospital.

Never use sticky bandages or other lotions, ointments, or creams to a first or second degree burn that you are treating at home unless the skin is injured. Use antibiotic ointment and re-bandage any broken blisters with lukewarm water and antibacterial soap.

When to Look for Help

If you are unsure about the severity of a burn, call 911 or go to the nearest medical facility. Every burn on a child, as well as any of the following conditions, need medical attention:

- Third-degree burns

- Second-degree burns that cover an area larger than the palm of a hand
- First-degree burns larger than a five-palm sized area
- Burns that totally round a leg or an arm.
- Any "mixed" pattern with varying degrees of burn
- Hand, foot, face, or genital area burns

First Aid Treatment for Severe Burns

Anybody who has been burned and is feeling weak, disoriented, feverish, chills, or shaking should visit a doctor right once. Always phone 911 in the case of significant burns before doing the following measures, keeping safety in mind, and if possible:

1. Put out the fire that produced the burn by spraying water on it or rolling the injured person on the ground while covering them with a heavy towel, coat, or blanket, if possible. Make sure no burning objects come into touch with the injured individual, but don't take off any burnt clothes.
2. Clear the airway, if necessary, then do the for ABCs as stated in Chapter 2 before beginning CPR.
3. Cool the burned area with running water while being careful not to overcool the injured individual while treating minor burns.
4. If you're transferring the person by yourself, cover the burned area with a dry, sterile blanket or a clean, nonfibrous material like a sheet rather than a blanket or towel since

fibers may stick to the person's burns. Avoid popping blisters or using creams, ointments, or lotions.

All second- and third-degree burns with a diameter of two inches or greater need rapid medical intervention.

First Aid Treatment for Minor Burns

Following these steps will allow you to treat small burns, first-degree burns, and moderate second-degree burns appropriately at home:

1. To avoid chemical burns, remove any clothes or jewelry that has encountered the chemical and the chemical source.
2. Cool the burn under running water, immerse it in cool water, or cover it with cold compresses for five to twenty minutes to relieve pain and prevent the burn from harming surrounding tissue. Cover used packs and avoided placing ice directly on the skin.
3. When a first-degree burn has fully cooled, use lotion or moisturizer to soothe and prevent drying it out.
4. Cover the burn with a loosely wrapped sterile gauze bandage if necessary to keep airflow and pressure off the burn while minimizing pain. Let the burn to heal exposed, if possible, without hurting the area, since minor burns heal more rapidly and completely when they are not covered.
5. Use over-the-counter pain relievers such as aspirin (for adults only), ibuprofen, naproxen, and acetaminophen as needed.

6. You may use small scissors that have been sterilized in alcohol to cut a tiny hole in any blisters that are highly sensitive and loaded with fluid. Cleanse them, as well as any burst blisters, thoroughly with antibacterial soap and warm water before rebandaging and applying antibiotic ointment.

Keep the region moist with skin lotion until minor burns heal, and then cover it with clothes or a UV-protective sunscreen for a year or so to minimize future sun exposure. Scarred regions may need ongoing sun protection. Most minor burns will heal without leaving scars if treated properly, which might take as little as a week or as long as a month.

> ***NOTE!***
>
> *Never use butter, ointment, grease, oil, or any other substance to treat a burn. Take care to remove any valuables and clothing from the burned area. Let medical workers to remove anything that is stuck to the burn. Submerge the burn in cool (not freezing) water to avoid heat damage to nearby tissues.*

Airway Burns

Airway burns are often severe. Inform the 911 operator as soon as possible that you suspect there has been an airway burn. If a person has burns on their head, neck, face, or other exposed parts, or if they have been on fire or in a confined space fire, they may have burns on their airways (where gases and air can become superheated). In these conditions, the airway may become significantly restricted, preventing the body from receiving adequate oxygen. Often, highly apparent signs of airway burning include:

- Singed nose hairs
- Swelling and actual burning of the mouth and tongue
- Soot around the nose and mouth
- Breathing difficulties
- Very hoarse voice

If a conscious individual exhibits signs of airway damage, administer brief sips of cool water to reduce swelling and adjust garments around the neck to let the person breathe more easily. Put the individual at ease until help arrives.

First Aid Treatment for Chemical Burns

Chemical burns are always serious and may even be lethal. Please remember that in all first-aid situations, the patient's personal safety comes first. After the implementation of safety precautions:

1. If you must leave the location, take steps to prevent being exposed to any harmful fumes or chemicals that may be there.
2. Make sure the area is well-ventilated and close any open chemical containers.
3. Call the Poison Control Center and 911 as soon as possible.

Although the first-aid approach for chemical burns is like that for heat-related burns, it is generally slower. After the first indications of intense stinging pain, blistering, peeling, swelling, and/or discoloration of the burn site usually emerge.

1. Remove any clothing items that may have been contaminated by the individual.
2. Wipe away any leftover dry chemicals from the body and begin pouring cold water over the burn for at least 20 minutes, or until help arrives.
3. Use disposable rubber gloves to protect yourself from contamination while attempting to avoid having the contaminated water you're dumping pool on or near you.

Chemical Eye Burns

Chemical eye burns may cause severe, irreversible, or complete damage of the eye. To minimize chemical burns, use gloves and avoid sprinkling more chemicals on oneself. Avoid touching your eye or trying to remove a contact lens that seems to be stuck in your eye (or let the injured person to do it).

The following methods are used to treat a chemical eye burn:

1. Begin by washing your eyes and continue for at least five minutes. At the workplace, go to the emergency eye-wash station and use sterile isotonic saline solution. If none of these options are available, use cold tap water. To clean your eye at home, go in the shower straight away while still wearing your clothing.

2. Try to keep your eyes as open as possible while rinsing them with running water or eye solution.
3. If you have alkali or hydrofluoric acid burns, keep washing until help arrives or you are taken to an emergency facility.

> ***NOTE!***
>
> *Children are often burnt by household chemicals because of alkali included in dishwashing detergent. Keep youngsters away from household cleaning materials, paints, solvents, and other potentially harmful items.*

Go through the product's label. Call your local Poison Control Center to find out what sort of chemical you were exposed to. The Poison Control Center may also advise you if you should seek medical assistance right now. If you experience any pain, tears, redness, irritation, vision loss, or are in doubt, go to an emergency room very away.

Sunburn

Sunburn hurts may be incapacitating, and increases your risk of getting skin cancer, however it seldom causes death. A sunburn is a kind of skin burn caused by ultraviolet (UV) radiation. It promotes skin irritation, premature aging, and wrinkles. Despite normal, limited exposure to UV radiation, which helps the skin produce vitamin D, any recent sun exposure and prior burns increase your risk.

VITAL!

Sunscreen should be applied 30 minutes before sun exposure for optimal efficacy. Moreover, despite what the label indicates, sunscreens must be reapplied generously after swimming, perspiring, and any sun exposure since they are not waterproof.

First Aid Treatment for Sunburn

Sunburn may be avoided by avoiding the sun, covering exposed skin, avoiding tanning beds, and wearing sunscreen with a high SPF (Sun Protection Factor). SPF assesses how long it takes to produce a skin reaction on protected and unprotected skin. In principle, SPF 30 permits you to stay out in the sun for thirty times longer than you would without sunscreen. However, this is rarely the case because people rarely apply sunscreen correctly and appropriately, and there is a limit to how much sun exposure is safe even when using sunscreen frequently.

To treat a sunburn, follow these steps:

- Use over-the-counter pain relievers for any discomfort.
- To treat light sunburn, apply a cold compress with milk and water or a cold compress with Burrows Solution, which is available at pharmacies.
- Use aloe plant juice or aloe-based lotions to moisturize.
- Bathe in warm water—not ice—but avoid bath salts, oils, and perfumes to prevent adverse symptoms.

- When using topical anesthetic medicines, avoid using lotions, shaving, or other skin-care items to prevent becoming allergic or sensitive to the therapy.
- While you are recuperating, avoid the sun and eat plenty of beverages.

If you have any major blistering, are dehydrated, or are suffering heat exhaustion, consult your doctor straight away.

CAUTION!

Sunburn may be reduced by using Sulfa medicines, antibiotics, tranquilizers, birth control pills, painkillers for arthritis, oral diabetic drugs, St. John's wort, medications for cancer, high blood pressure, and heart rhythm difficulties, as well as therapies for acne and other skin diseases.

Electrical Injuries

When a human comes into touch with an electrical energy source by mistake, an electric shock occurs, which may cause anything from a burn to a deadly or seriously disabling ailment. A person who has been shocked by electricity may have evident severe burns or may show no outward evidence of injury. An electrical shock may cause cardiac arrest. If you get a high-voltage shock or a shock that causes burns, go to the nearest emergency facility straight soon. A fast low-voltage shock, on the other hand, that does not cause any symptoms or skin burns does not need care or treatment. Children who get electric-current burns to the lips should see a doctor very once.

For all severe injuries, phone 911 and follow the emergency care guidelines in Chapter 2.

First Aid for Electrical Burns

Electrical burns may occur when a person's body is exposed to electricity. While mild burns are common at the entry and exit areas, you should be mindful that internal damage may run between the burns at these spots. There may be swelling and charring in both cases.

1. Call 911 immediately.
2. The individual might be unconscious, brain dead, or in cardiac arrest. Evaluate the unconscious person's breathing and pulse and start CPR if necessary.
3. If the victim is awake, splash cold water over the burns until help arrives, but never pour water near a live electrical source.

When approaching someone with a suspected electrical burn, be sure that contact with the electrical source has been severed and the current has been switched off.

Head Injury and Head Trauma

Slipping, tripping, and falling accidents kill thousands of people and leave millions permanently handicapped each year. Falls often result in broken bones, but falls may also result in more serious damage known as brain trauma or head injury.

In fact, head injuries from slipping, tripping, or falling are one of the leading causes of disability and death in both children and adults.

Head injuries may vary from mild to serious, and they can damage the skull and scalp. They may also have an impact on the brain, underlying tissues, and blood arteries in the skull. Depending on the severity of the head trauma, a head injury may also be referred to as a brain injury or traumatic brain injury (TBI). Concussions are brain injuries that may cause a loss of consciousness or awareness for a few minutes or hours. Contusions are brain injuries that cause bleeding and edema inside the brain at the site of the head's impact. A skull fracture is a break in the skull bone.

In head traumas caused by falling or a direct impact to the head, such as shaking a child, bruising and damage to the brain, tissue, and blood vessels occur from the brain jolting backward, striking the skull on one side, then rebounding to strike the other side. This shaking may cause tearing of tissues, blood vessels, and bodily tissues, resulting in internal bleeding, bruises, or brain enlargement.

Symptoms Of Head Injuries

Minor head injuries DO NOT need medical attention.

Minor head injuries will include the following symptoms:

- Headache
- Swollen area from a bump to small cuts in the scalp.

Moderate to severe head injuries symptoms will include:

- Vomiting
- Severe headache
- Blurry vision
- Loss of consciousness
- Confusion
- Sweating and pale skin
- Weakness on one side or area of the body
- Dizziness
- Inability or difficulty walking
- Slurred speech
- Deep cuts or lacerations in the scalp, foreign object penetrating the head, or an open wound in the head.

Deep scalp lacerations, an open head wound, or both. Also, there may be irritation and a loss of short-term memory, making it difficult to recollect the previous occurrence or occurrences with precision.

First Aid for Head Injuries

If you see any signs of a moderate-to-severe head injury, call 911 immediately. Mild head injuries may be treated and cared for at home, but if you are unclear of the severity of the head injury, immediately call your doctor or seek medical attention. In the case of bleeding beneath the scalp or "goose egg" damage outside the skull, use cold packs as soon as possible to reduce swelling. The eggs eventually mature and go on their own. Never apply ice directly to the skin; instead, use a clean towel to cover the region, a bag of frozen veggies wrapped in clean cloths, or store-bought chemical ice packs. Apply the therapy for 20 to 30 minutes at a period during the first 20 to 4 hours, roughly every 2 to 4 hours.

Mild injuries are often caused by falls from heights below the person's height that impact on soft surfaces such as carpets and DO NOT result in a loss of consciousness. Ice should be used to these injuries to minimize swelling while keeping a careful check on the patient. Bed rest with the head raised, water, and a mild pain reliever such as acetaminophen should be given as needed. As stated in Chapter 4, heal any minor wounds. A doctor should inspect any deep wounds for foreign items and hidden injuries. The wounds will also be cleaned, closed with stitches, staples, or glue, and a tetanus shot will be delivered if the injured individual hasn't had one in the preceding five to ten years.

VITAL!

To make an ice pack, combine two-thirds of a cup of water and one-third of a cup of 70% isopropyl alcohol in a plastic zip-top bag. This combination will solidify into slush. These packets may be made ahead of time and frozen for later use. When you have small children, use crushed ice in water instead of this combination since drinking it may be detrimental.

Headache and Head Pain

Tension headaches are the most frequent kind of headache, caused by tense and inflexible muscles in your shoulders, neck, scalp, and jaw. Stress, sorrow, or anxiety are the most common causes of these illnesses. Tension headaches may occur if you overwork, miss meals, drink alcohol, or DO NOT get enough sleep. Although migraines, cluster headaches, and sinus headaches are very common, it's important to be aware of lifestyle changes, relaxation techniques, and medicines you may use to cure your headaches. People have headaches for a variety of causes; however, they are less frequent and may be a symptom of a severe condition. Any sudden, severe headaches, headaches that worsen after a blow to the head, headaches accompanied by stiff necks, fevers, convulsions, a change in your regular pattern of headaches, or discomfort in your eyes or ears must be reported to your doctor.

Examining a Headache

You might be able to assist your doctor discover the source of your headache if you describe your headache symptoms and features as thoroughly as possible. This is referred to as presenting a "headache history." Provide your doctor the following information:

- Age when the headaches first started.
- How often do they happen?
- If you have one or more types of headaches
- Intensity of headaches

- Any known triggers such as events, meals, or drugs
- History of family headaches
- Symptoms that occur in-between headaches
- In the case that headaches hinder your ability to function
- If physical activity causes or aggravates a headache
- Any further information about the headache

Describe the location of the pain, how it feels (such as stabbing, pounding, or throbbing), the intensity of the pain on a scale of 1 (mild) to 10 (severe, resulting in crying), the duration of the headaches, whether they start suddenly without warning or with other symptoms, the time of day they typically occur, and whether you have vision changes, blind spots, or bright lights before the headache. Include any additional symptoms or warning signs, such as tiredness, nausea, sensitivity to light or noise, changes in appetite, attitude or behavior changes, and past headache therapy. Include any current drugs you are taking.

> ***NOTE!***
>
> *Most tension headaches may be treated with over the counter (OTC) medications such as aspirin (for adults only), ibuprofen, and acetaminophen. Take a pain reliever as soon as you notice a headache developing since, they function best when taken before the pain gets overwhelming.*

Women are more likely than men to suffer from migraines, and those who do may need prescription medication. A migraine's symptoms include pain that usually only affects one side of the head, nausea, vomiting, sensitivity to light or sound, and discomfort that worsens with frequent activity and may last anywhere from a few hours to 72 hours.

Cluster headaches affect just 1% of people and are characterized by abrupt, acute, or lingering pain on only one side of the head, as well as watery eyes and nasal congestion. One or more cluster headaches per day are common with these headaches throughout the period of two to twelve weeks. Cluster headaches, which often last 45 to 90 minutes, might trigger agitation, pacing, or rocking.

Rebound headaches are headaches caused by long-term use of any medication, and they may afflict anybody who regularly uses prescription medicines. The only way to treat rebound headaches is to reduce or discontinue the medicine that is generating the headaches. Headaches may last anywhere from five minutes to 48 hours after indulging in a certain activity, such as exercise, sex, or coughing fits. This kind of headache might suggest high blood pressure.

First Aid Treatment for Headaches

When migraines arise owing to increased sensitivity to light and sound, try to relax in a quiet, dark place and apply hot or cold compresses to your head or neck. A little bit of coffee and massage treatment may be beneficial at times. Most headaches are moderate and manageable and can be treated over-the-counter painkiller. If your headache persists or worsens, see your doctor. For a sudden and severe headache caused by:

- Rash
- Stiff neck
- Fever
- Mental confusion
- Dizziness
- Change in vision.
- Loss of balance
- Weakness
- Seizures
- Difficulty speaking
- Numbness

Get medical attention if you have a headache that:

- Is a severe case of caused by a recent respiratory infection or sore throat.
- Starts or worsens after a head injury, bump, or fall.
- If you are fifty or older and experiencing new types of pain.
- It is painful.
- Just one reddened eye is affected.
- Worsens During the course of the day.
- Continues for many days.

A cold shower may help relieve tension headaches by lowering body temperature. Caffeine may be used to prevent and treat migraines because it constricts blood vessels. When you get a headache, your blood vessels dilate. Caffeine should be avoided on a regular basis since it might cause headaches that return after use. To prevent and manage headaches, do the following steps:

- Keep a headache log to help you identify the cause of your headaches, such as foods and triggers in your environment.
- Avoid certain triggers including alcoholic drinks, pickled foods, MSG, caffeine, smoked meats and cheeses, loud noises, and bright lights.
- To stay healthy, eat a low-fat, high-complex-carb diet.
- Consume one cup of drink for every twenty pounds of body weight each day to stay hydrated.
- Have modest, frequent meals to prevent low blood sugar.
- Mild exercises such as yoga, tai chi, or swimming should be part of a regular fitness regimen.
- Have a regular sleeping pattern to get seven to nine hours of sleep every night.

CAUTION!

Some headaches are symptoms of serious underlying problems. If you have a severe headache that worsens despite rest and over-the-counter pain medicines, or if it is accompanied by other symptoms such as a fever, stiff neck, rash, double vision, weakness, disorientation, seizure, numbness, or trouble speaking, seek immediate medical assistance.

Abdominal Pain

Abdominal pain may be felt in several ways, including burning, cramping, stabbing, throbbing, spasming, and intense discomfort under the ribs, above the pelvic bone, and around the flanks on either side. While skin and abdominal-wall muscles may produce discomfort in this area, abdominal pain is often associated with pain from internal organs such as the stomach, large and small intestines, appendix, colon, liver, gall bladder, and pancreas. Referred pain occurs when discomfort felt in the abdomen is really caused by the lower lungs, kidneys, uterus, or ovaries.

Inflammation, organ strain or swelling, or a decrease of blood supply to an organ are all reasons that contribute to stomach pain. Irritable bowel syndrome is one condition in which stomach pain may arise without any of these other causes (IBS). Although the cause of IBS is unknown, it may be caused by abnormal contractions of the intestinal muscles (spasm) or too sensitive nerves that cause pain in the intestines. Some stomach pain is deemed an emergency, such as appendicitis, while others, such as diverticulitis or colitis, are chronic. Every episode of stomach pain should be evaluated by a doctor since it might be serious, even deadly.

To properly express the pain and symptoms to your doctor, the following symptoms should be documented in children:

- The duration of pain, particularly pain that lasts longer than twenty-four hours.
- Where the pain is located and any pain outside the center of the abdomen.
- Features of the child's appearance, such as paleness, sweat, fatigue, and listlessness.
- Experiencing nausea and vomiting for more than twenty-four hours or having red colored vomit.
- If there is blood in the school or if the diarrhea lasts for than seventy-two hours.
- Presence or absence of fever.
- Groin pain (may indicate blood supply being cut Off from a testicle twisting on itself)
- Bladder problems
- Abdominal pain in addition to any rash

After speaking with or having your doctor examine you, continue to monitor your child's symptoms and notify them if anything changes or if there has been no improvement. Also, bear in mind that, depending on their age, children may be reluctant to report problems.

First Aid for Treatment Abdominal Pain

The occurrence of intense abdominal pain may suggest the existence of a serious sickness. You may need to describe your pain to the doctor. This is readily understood if you imagine that 0 represents no pain and 10 represents misery so acute that you are weeping, and your face is distorted in a grimace.

Indicate if the pain is intense or moderate, burning, pressure-like, jabbing, transitory, continuous, or cramp-like. Take note of any fever, chills, sweats, rectal bleeding, loss of appetite, diarrhea, weight loss, constipation, nausea, or fatigue. Treating minor abdominal pain requires the following steps:

- Rest
- Taking a hot bath or using a heating pad
- Antacids, both prescription and over the counter (but avoid aspirin or ibuprofen, as these drugs can make some types of stomach pain and conditions worse)
- Consume a regular food and lots of water as tolerated.

See your doctor if you have any of the following symptoms: persistent discomfort, fever, vomiting, vaginal bleeding, loss of consciousness, chest pain, or any serious symptoms.

Diagnosis of the reason of stomach pain may be difficult, and it often requires many medical visits and tests, such as blood tests, radiographic examinations, and endoscopic procedures.

Nausea and Vomiting

Everyone experiences nausea and vomiting from time to time, which usually pass quickly and may be managed at home with nausea drugs and fluid replenishment to avoid dehydration. Fluid rehydration may also help rectify any electrolyte imbalances, which may help halt the vomiting.

First Aid for Treating Nausea and Vomiting

Follow these steps to get rid of nausea and vomiting:

1. Hydrate with clear liquids (clear soup, broth, juice, herbal tea), beginning with little sips and gradually increasing to eight ounces at a time, or one ounce at a time, or less for children.
2. Avoid milk and other dairy products that may cause nausea and vomiting.
3. If you can stomach clear liquids, begin eating soft, basic meals like oatmeal and yogurt.
4. Provide rehydrating oral liquids to children, such as Pedialyte and Rehydrate.
5. Coffee, tea, fruit juice, and sports drinks are not adequate substitutes for fluids and electrolytes.
6. Avoid drinking plain water since it lacks electrolytes and may promote an electrolyte imbalance in a dehydrated body, which might lead to seizures.

If you have trouble swallowing drinks, you should see a doctor so that an IV may be administered to rehydrate you.

> ***NOTE!***
>
> *The World Health Organization has issued this advice for fluid rehydration. One quart of clean or bottled water should be mixed with two tablespoons of sugar or honey, respectively (honey should only be used for children one year of age and older). Use it in the same way you would any other rehydrating beverage.*

Asthma Attack

Asthma affects the lungs' breathing pathways (bronchioles) due to chronic inflammation. Because of this inflammation, an asthmatic's airways become very sensitive to particular "triggers," causing the passages to expand and fill with mucus. As a result, the muscles in the breathing passages contract and spasm (bronchospasm), further narrowing the airway channels and making it more difficult to expel air from the lungs. Wheezing, difficulty breathing, pain or tightness in the chest, anxiety, coughing, choking feeling, sweating, an increase in heart rate, and persistent, spasmodic coughing that is typically worse at night are all signs of an asthma attack.

If you have asthma, you must learn to control the illness and be aware of the likelihood of an attack whenever you are exposed to anything that causes an attack in you. Although asthma cannot be cured, it is controllable, particularly if discovered early and treated promptly. Always follow your doctor's treatment instructions and visit them on a regular basis. Notify your doctor if your symptoms change or worsen, or if any medication side effects arise. Asthma symptoms and attacks are treated with the objective of avoiding and treating them, particularly those severe enough to need a trip to the ER or hospitalization.

You might have an asthma attack at any moment. The following are some of the markers to look for to discover whether your symptoms are becoming worse:

- Sweating
- You're breathing so fiercely that it's tough for you to speak.
- The skin surrounding your ribs is dimpling as we breathe out via your abdominal muscles.
- The lips and fingernails are blue in color.
- The nostrils begin to widen as you breathe in.
- Even after being given emergency medications, the patient continues to wheeze, breathe deeply, and cough.

First Aid Treatment for Asthma

Anybody suffering from asthma must be constantly aware of her symptoms, avoid triggers, and understand how to regulate her symptoms. Use these steps to manage asthma attacks:

- Find out what your triggers are and how to prevent them.
- Quit smoking cigarettes and doing drugs at the same time.

- Over-the-counter inhalers are not recommended since they are fast-acting drugs that are unlikely to prevent an asthma attack and may have harmful side effects.
- Avoid using non-prescription medications, herbs, or nutritional supplements unless you've discussed them with your doctor, since some may have unpleasant side effects and others may interfere with your prescription drugs.
- Avoid taking more asthma medication than is required, since this may be dangerous.

If you experience an asthma attack, take your prescription rescue medication (inhaled beta-agonist) twice, one minute between each puff (OR as directed by your doctor), and call your doctor if you DO NOT feel better straight away. If you are currently taking oral or inhaled steroids and your treatments are not working, you must notify your doctor. Since your doctor's advice are just broad guidelines, always follow them exactly.

If you are experiencing a severe asthma attack and are having difficulty breathing, call 911 immediately. DO NOT try to drive by yourself.

Chapter 7

Major Emergencies

Basic first aid is required for many accidents and situations, but others may need more examination and expert treatment. A little cut is usually easy to cure, but a large, possibly lethal trauma, such as a gunshot wound, needs greater care. You never know when you'll be the first to detect a multiple-car crash, an accident that may have resulted in spinal injury, or a family member suffering from a stroke. To minimize future injury and contribute to the preservation of lives, it is critical to learn how to detect the seriousness of all injuries and to respond quickly, attentively, and effectively.

Bleeding

Bleeding occurs when a blood vessel or vessels are damaged. External bleeding may occur because of a cut or wound, but internal bleeding can occur when the skin is not broken but internal blood vessels are affected. There are three kinds of bleeding based on the type of vessel that is damaged. The bright red blood that explodes in a jet with each heartbeat is arterial bleeding produced by damaged arteries. Venous bleeding is caused by damaged veins and resulting in dark red blood loss that may be less severe but may flow continually. Capillary hemorrhage, which generally results in just a modest loss of blood, is generated by tiny blood vessels present throughout the body. The depth of a cut, the amount of bleeding, the time it takes to stop the bleeding, and the kind of blood vessels affected are all elements that indicate the severity of an injury. Any bleeding injury poses the risk of infection, particularly if a foreign object becomes trapped in the wound.

NOTE!

An adult of average size may safely lose one pint of blood since their total blood volume is less than 10 quarts. Any excessive blood loss, often known as shock, may result in a dramatic reduction in blood pressure, general weakness, confusion, and sweating.

First Aid Treatment for Bleeding

While blood loss is rarely life-threatening, some individuals react negatively to the sight of blood, causing them to behave oddly, feel dizzy, or even go into shock.

1. Even if it means engaging in mundane talk, try to keep the individual as calm as possible.
2. Remember to observe the person's ABCs, and if necessary, have him lie down and manage for shock (see Chapter 2).
3. Apart from wounds produced by a foreign object such as glass or those with protruding bone, most bleeding wounds should be treated with direct pressure. Push down hard on

these wounds. Keep the injured body part above the level of the heart on either side of the item.

Handling Severe Bleeding

Arterial bleeding may be dangerous and is often difficult to stop. The primary and most effective technique of bleeding control is direct pressure. This is what you should do:

1. Place something clean and hygienic over the area and tape it down or wrap something over the wound that is just tight enough to stop the flow.
2. If the bleeding does not cease, place another bandage over the previous one or apply direct pressure to the incision as illustrated below.
3. Never take a dressing off after it has been applied to a major wound.
4. Raise an injured arm, leg, or head above the level of the heart to help stop the bleeding.
5. If you suspect a broken bone (fracture), don't raise, or move the afflicted area of the body until you've applied a splint as indicated in Chapter 9 and are certain that doing so won't cause more harm.

When direct pressure and elevation are not stopping the bleeding, you may use indirect pressure by applying pressure at the proper pressure point. You may regulate blood flow in certain areas by pressing an artery against an underlying bone with your fingers, thumb, or heel of the hand. Use pressure points with caution since you risk harming an extremity if the nearby pressure does not offer adequate blood flow. Never apply pressure to the carotid pressure points in the neck since doing so may reduce or halt blood supply to the brain and result in cardiac arrest.

The groin and upper arm are the two basic pressure points that are often used. The pressure point is the front, center region of the groin crease, which sends the bulk of blood to each leg. The female oral artery begins in the lower abdomen and goes down into the thigh. Finding the pulse in the inner thigh and pressing it up against the pelvic bone will help you find this artery.

The brachial artery may be in the upper, inner arm, directly below the bicep and halfway between the shoulder and elbow. Apply pressure on the inside of the arm, over the bone, using your fingers or thumb. If there is significant bleeding in the lower leg or thigh, place the injured person on her back and kneel. Put pressure on the female oral artery point on the side opposite the affected leg by squeezing the heel of your hand there and pushing forward. If the bleeding is still uncontrollable, push the artery with the flat surface of your fingertips. You may apply more pressure to your fingers by pushing down with the heel of your other hand.

If alternative means of reducing bleeding are inadequate, never use tourniquets because they might cause tissue damage and limb loss. You may use a strap, belt, necktie, towel, or any other piece of material that is six to seven layers thick and three or more inches wide. Never use wire or anything that might nick the skin.

To use a tourniquet, perform these steps:

1. Place the tourniquet such that there are two or more inches of intact skin between it and the wound while maintaining the right pressure point.
2. Putting a pad or gauze roll over the artery.
3. Tie a half-knot (the first step in tying a shoelace) on the upper surface after wrapping the tourniquet twice around the injured limb.
4. Complete the knot by inserting a small stick or other object on the midway point (square knot).
5. When the bleeding has stopped, slowly twist the stick to tighten it before fastening it.
6. DO NOT cover the tourniquet.
7. Draw a "T" on the person's forehead using a marker (like lipstick) to denote that a tourniquet was placed and when it was administered.

CAUTION!

Never use a tourniquet as a last option to stop serious bleeding, and only on the extremities. After a tourniquet has been applied, DO NOT loosen, or remove it since doing so may dislodge clots, resulting in more blood loss, shock, and death.

Internal Bleeding / Blunt Trauma

Internal bleeding is more difficult to identify and treat than external bleeding, which is generally obvious. Losing blood may result in dangerously low blood pressure due to insufficient blood volume, a condition called as hypovolemic shock, which can be fatal if ignored. It may also result in inadequate blood supply to tissues and organs.

> ***VITAL!***
>
> *Call your doctor immediately if you feel bleeding from anybody orifice, including the mouth, ears, nose, or rectum. This is an indicator of internal bleeding, a severe sickness that requires immediate medical treatment.*

If you're looking for a unique way to express yourself, here is the place to be. Occurring outside the uterus and requiring prompt medical treatment). Normally, blunt trauma, powerful force, such as in a car accident, or puncture wounds, such as knife or gunshot wounds, result in serious internal bleeding. Internal bleeding should be considered if there are shock symptoms.

The following are the most prevalent signs of internal bleeding:

- Rapid breathing (tachypnea)
- Nausea and vomiting
- Excessive thirst
- Anxiety and restlessness
- Bruises (contusions), which may suggest deeper damage.

- Blood in stool, or black and tar like looking stool.
- Any bruise or discoloration at the area of injury
- Rapid, weak pulse (tachycardia)
- Pale ashen or skin turning blue.
- Cold and clammy skin
- Severe headache
- Decreased level of consciousness
- Vomiting dark red (resemblance to coffee grounds)
- Swelling, distended (bloated) abdomen.
- Blood in the urine

First Aid Treatment for Internal Bleeding

To control internal bleeding, follow these steps:

1. To reduce pain and swelling, use a cold pack or ice pack wrapped with a towel to bruises.
2. If there is no chest injury, call 911 and position the injured individual with their legs up.
3. In the case of a chest injury, elevate the head and torso and keep the patient warm until help arrives.
4. Manage shock as mentioned in Chapter 2.
5. DO NOT let the individual to ingest food, drinks, or drugs only if a doctor has ordered you to do so.

VITAL!

If the injured person shows any of these symptoms, such as chest pain, difficulty breathing, or bruising, grazes, or discoloration in the chest area, you should be on the alert for internal bleeding and be prepared to give shock.

Penetrating Trauma

Gunshot wounds were formerly only seen on television, but the sad but true reality is that these potentially lethal wounds are becoming increasingly frequent in everyday life. If you're looking for a unique way to express yourself, here is the place to be. Penetrating trauma includes gunshot wounds and injuries caused by knife stabbing.

Penetrating trauma occurs when an instrument pierces the skin or enters the body's tissue, as in gunshot and knife wounds. The severity of a penetrating injury frequently rises with the speed (velocity) of penetration, which may range from superficial punctures to penetration of major physiological systems.

First Aid Treatment for Penetrating Trauma

Gunshot wounds are often treated the same as other puncture wounds such as knife wounds. Remember to prioritize your safety and the safety of anybody who may be assisting you. Knowing that a penetrating injury may be life-threatening is critical for gauging its severity. This is determined by the kind of item used, the location and depth of penetration, and the number of wounds. Knives and ice picks create low-energy injuries since they are employed at close range, yet one significant cut from a large knife to the center of a person's chest, neck, or head is certainly considerably worse than multiple minor wounds to an arm or leg.

Consider spinal injuries in the case of any piercing head, chest, or neck injuries, OR a wound that causes a person to fall, and stabilize and protect the neck by holding the head firmly in place in line with the body. Assess for ABCs and manage in accordance with the principles in Chapter 2.

In treating chest wounds, keep an eye out for any potentially concerning symptoms, such as shortness of breath, blue skin, back discomfort, or the sound of airflow sucking or hissing through the puncture hole, sometimes known as a sucking chest wound.

Keep an eye out for any signs of "flail chest," which happens when a piece of the chest contracts when a person inhales while the rest of the chest expands, and when a person exhales while the rest of the chest contracts.

Use the following procedures to treat a sucking chest wound:

1. If clothing is stuck to the wound in a chemical environment, DO NOT attempt to clean or remove it.
2. If at all feasible, cover the wound with the person's hand while applying an occlusive dressing. This may be any kind of plastic wrap, aluminum foil, or duct tape and should be put two inches beyond the border of the wound to prevent it

from being dragged back in. After that, apply adhesive tape to seal the repair.

3. Once the user exhales, air will flow out of the chest cavity and leave through the patch's open border since only three sides should be taped. When the user inhales, the patch sticks to the skin, preventing more air from entering the chest cavity (this method of patching helps to reinflate a collapsed lung).
4. Firmly put a larger dressing. Rolling the individual on their damaged side until aid arrives while covering the patch so that it doesn't impede breathing.
5. Treat a flailed chest injury with a thick, bulky dressing.

Examine your pulse at the neck or carotid, wrist, groin, feminine, and finally. If you can't feel a pulse in the carotid artery, you should start CPR. Move the wounded person only if doing so jeopardizes his or her safety; until aid comes, place unconscious persons in the recovery position, as instructed in Chapter 2.

Don't wipe up any blood on clothing, vehicle seats, or the ground since first responders need it to calculate the amount of blood lost before reporting to the emergency room. Also, in situations of any violent crime, including domestic abuse, DO NOT dispose of or destroy any further evidence, such as plainly stained or not soiled underwear or blood-soaked clothes.

Be in mind that mishaps involving guns and other weapons might endanger rescuers and first responders. Above everything, be safe.

Use common sense. If you become harmed, you are no assistance to the injured person. If you are convinced that a gun is involved, call 911 straight away. When a person is transported to a hospital in an ambulance within 10 minutes after being shot, they have a better chance of survival.

Spinal Cord Injury

Since spinal cord injuries are often associated with dangerous events such as avalanches, rockslides, and car accidents, it is critical that you assess the scene's safety before offering help. After doing the ABCs, phone 911 and determine the injured person's level of consciousness by asking them their name, where they are, what time it is, and if they remember what happened. Incorrect answers to the first three questions are indicative of a brain injury and may also suggest spinal cord damage.

It is critical to evaluate any signs of drug or alcohol use, as well as any other conditions that are causing the individual enough suffering that they are unable to ignore their spinal disc damage. If pink coloration does not return two seconds after pressure is released from a fingernail on each hand and toenail on each foot, this may suggest a spinal injury-related loss of circulation. Ask the guy to move his fingers and toes; limb stiffness or immobility are indicators of a spinal injury. Numbness OR tingling when gently compressing the fingers, as well as these symptoms, suggest possible spinal injury.

If you are doubtful, always assume a spinal cord damage exists. Maintain your posture above the injured person's head while supporting their neck firmly but gently with one hand on either side of the head. If you need to transfer the individual for any reason, follow the instructions in Chapter 2. Support the injured person's neck until help arrives.

Stroke

Since brain cells begin to die within minutes of blood supply to the brain ending, strokes are a medical emergency that requires immediate treatment. The most frequent kind of stroke occurs when a blood clot travels to and stops a blood artery in the brain from any part of the body. Hemorrhagic stroke is the second kind of stroke, and it happens when a blood artery in the brain rupture and bleeds into the brain. Transient ischemic attacks (TIA), also known as tiny strokes, occur when the brain's blood supply is suddenly disturbed, often for one minute but less than five minutes, and they DO NOT affect the brain due to their brief duration. TIA is a significant stroke predictor.

The warning signals of a stroke or transient ischemic attack are abrupt and include:

- The face, arm, or leg may feel numb or weak, particularly on one side only.
- Confusion
- Difficulty comprehending or speaking.

- Vision problems in one or both eyes
- Having difficulty walking
- Dizziness
- Coordination and balance issues
- Severe headache for no apparent cause

First Aid Treatment for Stroke

If you see any of these symptoms, call 911 immediately because prompt medical attention may prevent a stroke from becoming fatal or incapacitating. Then do the following:

1. Check for ABCs and start CPR if necessary.
2. Unconscious persons should be put in the recovery position, as explained in Chapter 2.
3. Gently lay the individual down while supporting his head and shoulders with pillow or folded clothes.
4. Don't give him any food or drink.
5. Assure the person that help is on the way.

Poisoning

A person may be poisoned by injecting, inhaling, coming into touch with, or swallowing a harmful item. According to the CDC, there are approximately 2.5 million reported poisonings in the United States each year. A product that does not carry a warning label is not necessarily safe. Although signs of poisoning may take some time to appear, if you feel someone you know has been poisoned, seek emergency medical assistance for that individual immediately.

Certain ancient objects, such as medications (for example, an aspirin overdose), old cleaning products, carbon monoxide, some old plants, paints, pesticides, chemicals, and even some foods, may be toxic if a human mistakenly comes into touch with them. Symptoms might vary based on the scenario, but they may include:

- Cough
- Confusion
- Chest pain
- Bluish lips
- Abdominal pain
- Drowsiness
- Dizziness
- Blurred vision.
- Difficulty breathing
- Diarrhea
- Nausea and vomiting
- Muscle twitching
- Heart palpitations
- Headache
- Fever
- Loss of consciousness
- Stupor
- Skin rash and burns
- Seizures
- Tingling and numbness

- Weakness
- Unusual breath odor

First Aid Treatment for Poisoning

If you suspect someone is poisoning, take these steps:

1. After verifying for ABCs, phone 911, begin rescue breathing and CPR if necessary, and then dial 1-800-222-1222 for Poison Control Center support.
2. Try to identify the poison and avoid making the victim vomit until instructed to do so by the poison control center (note that parents should not use syrup of ipecac at home anymore).
3. If the individual vomits on their own, open the airway, but first wrap a towel over your fingers before clearing your mouth and throat.
4. If the individual begins to have a seizure, laying them down carefully on a soft surface may help avoid further injury. Maintain the airway open by tilting the head to one side rather than restraining the victim.
5. Until help arrives, roll unconscious persons onto their left side in the recovery position (see Chapter 2).
6. If poison has been poured on the victim, remove their clothing, and wash their skin with water.

> ***VITAL!***
>
> *Anybody who becomes unwell for no apparent cause and is found near a furnace, vehicle, or fire, or in a poorly ventilated area, must be evaluated for poisoning. In such circumstances, contact the Poison Control Center.*

If you suspect inhalation poisoning, call 911 immediately and remove the individual from the danger zone of the gas, fumes, or smoke only if it is safe to do so. Holding your breath or covering your nose and mouth with a damp towel might help clear the air of pollutants. All of the windows should be opened.

Drug Overdose

A drug overdose occurs when more medication is taken more often or in bigger doses than the body can process. Some overdoses are accidental, while others are unintended. If prescription medications are coupled with illegal drugs and alcohol, overdosing is also a risk. The following overdose symptoms vary depending on the drug used:

- Small (pinpoint) or enlarged pupils.
- Low or high temperature
- Loss of coordination
- Abdominal breathing
- Slurred speech
- Loss of consciousness
- Hallucinations and delusions

- Drowsiness
- Sweating
- Red and flushed face
- Death

First Aid Treatment for Drug Overdose

If you suspect someone is suffering from a drug overdose, give the following first aid measures:

1. Check for ABCs and begin CPR if necessary.
2. Manage for seizures and shock.
3. The unconscious person should be put in the recovery position.
4. Any major or life-threatening symptoms, concerns about someone's safety, or thoughts of self-harm should be reported to 911.

DO NOT try to make the individual vomit. Call the PoisOn Control Center even if the individual seems to be OK. Inspect pill bottles and other medical supplies. to make an attempt to understand what the individual has taken in order to present medical personnel with proper information and the bottles or paraphernalia.

Dial 911 to report hostile or irrational behavior and to safeguard your own safety. Instead of expecting someone who is taking drugs to be rational or attempting to argue with her, call for help. Keep your emotions and ideas apart from your actions; all that is necessary is that you administer first aid; you don't even need to know why.

Near Drowning

Suffocation (severe oxygen deprivation) caused by immersion in water is considered near drowning if it does not result in death. When the occurrence results in death, it is referred to as a drowning. The following are the signs of a near-drowning:

- Alert but reluctant to sleep.
- The person is not breathing or is gasping for air, coughing, or wheezing.
- Vomiting
- The lips and ears are both blue (cyanosis)
- A pale appearance
- Skin that is cold

First Aid Treatment for Near Drowning

The following measures should be taken in the case of a near drowning:

1. If the individual is unconscious, start rescue breathing as indicated in Chapter 2 as soon as possible, preferably while the person is still in the water.
2. If at all feasible, have someone else phone 911 while you begin your rescue breathing.
3. After ensuring a safe landing, place the victim on his back, resume rescue breathing, and begin CPR if necessary.

Since the water comes from the stomach rather than the lungs, the individual must be rotated with a log roll for it to flow through their lips. Another risk is vomiting.

> ***NOTE!***
>
> *Several near-drowning events have had beneficial outcomes. It is possible to survive a forty-minute submersion with the proper rescue and treatment, and many people who get CPR and specialist care recover completely.*

Even if you believe the individual has been immersed for an extended amount of time, doing CPR and/or rescue breathing immediately will increase the odds of life and lessen the likelihood and severity of any brain damage. Make an attempt to stabilize and mobilize the neck to prevent exacerbating any spinal damage. Remove any wet clothes, wrap him in warm blankets, and transport him to the hospital if the individual is still aware, regardless of how quickly you revive him or how well he feels.

The length of submersion, water temperature (older-water accidents may have a better outcome), the person's age (children have better outcomes than adults), and how quickly resuscitation begins are the factors that have the greatest impact on a person's survival without permanent brain and lung damage. If a person almost drowns while drinking alcohol, their chances of dying or suffering brain or lung damage increase.

Carbon Monoxide Poisoning

Carbon monoxide is a colorless, flavorless, and odorless poisonous gas that may cause fatigue, headaches, and dizziness, and can even kill you in large amounts. When there is carbon monoxide in the air, oxygen-carrying cells transport the gas instead of oxygen, becoming saturated with it and unable to give the cells with the necessary levels of oxygen. For this reason, installing carbon monoxide detectors to warn of dangerous amounts is critical.

Because homes are often poorly aired and tightly sealed up from previous owners, most carbon monoxide poisoning incidents occur at night during the winter months. Carbon-monoxide gas is produced when carbon-containing compounds are completely burned in fireplaces, space heaters, forced-air gas furnaces, appliances, and motor vehicles. You are also at risk if your home has any non-electric equipment, such as a gas stove or water heater, or if it has a connected garage.

Symptoms of carbon monoxide poisoning include:

- Chest pain
- Difficulty moving
- Inability to concentrate.
- Dizziness and lightheadedness
- Weakness
- Irritability and lethargy in infants
- Coma

- Seizure
- Shortness of breath
- Headache
- Nausea

NOTE!

Only a carbon monoxide detector can ensure that you are not inhaling harmful chemicals while awake. Most retail outlets and hardware stores offer them at reasonable prices.

First Aid Treatment for Carbon Monoxide Poisoning

The following measures should be performed in the case of carbon monoxide poisoning:

1. If you wake up and notice symptoms of carbon monoxide poisoning, immediately slump to the ground and crawl to an escape.
2. If you are unable to safely evacuate anybody trapped within the structure by yourself, call 911. Avoid trying to rescue anybody who does not have the proper oxygen-delivery masks.
3. Make sure you're upwind of the home and get some fresh air as soon as possible.
4. Loosen any clothes that is too tight around your waist and neck.

5. If a person loses consciousness after entering, keep an open airway and begin CPR or rescue breathing as stated in Chapter 2.

Even if you feel well after being exposed to carbon monoxide, call 911 to receive an accurate evaluation and, if required, oxygen.

Chapter 8

Common Illnesses

Fever may accompany common ailments such as the cold or flu, causing you to miss work or social commitments or putting you out of action for a short period of time. Some events, such as nosebleeds and black eyes, are less painful but much more frightening. Learning how to deal with, treat, and prevent these conditions may also help you avoid larger problems in some circumstances, in addition to assisting you in managing the dread and worry that certain common injuries cause.

Fever

Fever is one of the body's defensive systems against many bacteria and viruses that prefer to live at the body's usual temperature of 98.6°F. By boosting the body's temperature and stimulating the immune system, the body strives to make it more difficult for certain kinds of invaders to survive. Mild fevers vary between 98.8°F and 100.8°F, mild to moderate fevers between 101°F and 103°F, and severe fevers between 104°F and higher. Fever may be caused by a variety of circumstances, including hot temperatures, vaccinations, bacterial and viral diseases, excessive sun exposure, and allergies. A fever is often associated with symptoms such as a heated face, sweating, lack of appetite, nausea, vomiting, bodily aches, constipation, and diarrhea. High fevers may sometimes be followed by delirium and convulsions.

NOTE!

Any oral temperature over 105°F is potentially deadly and requires immediate medical attention. Children should be treated similarly to adults for a cold or the flu, with non-aspirin over-the-counter fever medications such as children's or infant's acetaminophen or ibuprofen, according to the label.

Taking a Temperature

Most thermometers now include digital readouts for ear canal, underarm (axillary), and even mouth readings. Always read the directions to discover what the thermometer's beeps signify and when to read the temperature. Glass mercury thermometers are no longer recommended due to the dangers of mercury exposure or consumption.

Before taking a child's temperature rectally, you should:

1. Add some petroleum jelly or similar lubricant to the thermometer's bulb. The child should be positioned on her stomach.
2. Carefully insert the thermometer one and a half to one inch into the rectum.
3. Hold the child still for three minutes while holding the thermometer; don't let go.

4. Remove the thermometer and read it according to the manufacturer's instructions.

When taking an oral temperature is not possible or may be problematic, anyone of any age may take a rectal temperature.

Insert the thermometer's bulb end under the tongue, keep it there for the specified period of time (usually three minutes), then remove it and record the reading.

The most accurate way to take a temperature is not under the arm (axillary), but an oral thermometer may be used for an armpit reading if necessary. Oral readings are generally one degree lower than axillary readings. Place the thermometer under the arm with the arm down, while holding the arms across the chest. Remove your thermometer, wait five minutes, or the period specified by the manufacturer, and then take the temperature. If any of the following apply, get medical attention:

- Babies over the age of three months with a rectal temperature of at least 100.4°F or higher, even if no other symptoms exist.
- Infants older than three months with a fever of 102°F or higher
- Infants with lower-than-average temperatures or internal temperatures less than 97°F
- Children above the age of two who have been feverish for more than a day.

- Toddlers and older children with a fever lasting longer than three days.
- Children with fever after being left in a hot car or heated conditions: seek immediate medical assistance.
- Adults who have had a fever for more than three days or a temperature of more than 103°F.

If you have any of the following symptoms, contact your doctor straight away:

- Skin rashes
- Swelling of the throat (especially severe swelling)
- Severe headache
- Mental confusion
- Stiff neck / pain when bending the head forward or not being able to bend the neck forward.
- Sudden unusual sensitivity to bright light
- Excessive listlessness or irritability
- Chest pain or breathing difficulties.
- Continual vomiting
- Abdominal pain or pain during urination
- Any other symptoms of concern

The First Aid Treatment for Fever

If you have a fever, follow these steps:

1. A thermometer is used to measure the temperature.
2. Excess clothing and blankets must be removed.

3. DO NOT overheat the room.
4. Provide sponge baths in lukewarm water.
5. Stay hydrated by drinking plenty of water (watch for light-colored urine often, indicating a person is well hydrated).
6. Acetaminophen should be taken as directed on the package to reduce fever.

DO NOT:

- Give aspirin to somebody with fever.
- Rub rubbing alcohol to your skin or soak in it.

See your healthcare provider if you have any irregular breathing patterns, trouble breathing, stiff neck, disorientation, rashes, chronic sore throats, nausea, diarrhea, painful urination, or seizures. Adults with fevers under 102°F should not take any medication unless expressly advised to do so by their doctor. For fevers of 102°F or higher, only adults sixteen and older should use over-the-counter medications such as acetaminophen, ibuprofen, and aspirin.

Febrile Seizures

Children may have febrile seizures (convulsions), which are often caused by an illness that produces a rapid increase in body temperature. These seizures often last just a few minutes, yet they surprise and frighten parents. Despite their terrifying and threatening look, these seizures are often harmless and DO NOT suggest a long-term or chronic problem. A seizure will often begin before a fever or illness is even diagnosed. febrile seizures affect 2-

4 percent of children aged six months to five years. Although febrile seizures are extremely frequent and largely harmless, you should seek medical attention if you experience any, particularly if the underlying cause of the fever has to be addressed. To prevent febrile seizures, treat fevers in children who are prone to them as soon as they appear.

First Aid Treatment for Febrile Seizures

A febrile seizure may cause significant shaking or muscular stiffness, as well as eyelid rolling. Fever is often higher than 102°F, and it is accompanied by additional symptoms such as loss of consciousness, jerking or shaking of both arms and legs, rolling of the eyes back in the head, trouble breathing, peeing on demand, vomiting, and crying or weeping. Simple febrile seizures, which may last anywhere from a few seconds to fifteen minutes before terminating on their own, are the most common kind of seizure. To avoid febrile seizures, do the following steps:

1. Remove anything sharp or hard from the area.
2. Place the child on a soft surface (such as a bed or carpet), put him on his side to keep the airway open, and place a padded jacket or pillow under his head to protect the airway in the event of vomiting.
3. Remove any glasses and loosen any tight or restrictive clothes.

4. Have a look at your watch. Attempt to time the seizure and pay attention to any warning signs, such as a twitching or moving body part, so you can notify your doctor.
5. Call 911 A seizure lasting more than five minutes, two or more seizures, seizures followed by vomiting, respiratory problems, or considerable exhaustion after a seizure are all symptoms of febrile seizures.
6. After regaining consciousness, reassure the child and then call or visit your doctor as required.

DO NOT:

- Try putting anything in the mouth or holding the tongue.
- Try to restrain then child, rather, turn his head to the side so that his tongue or any vomit will not impede his airway.
- Try to cool down a fever during seizure by trying to cool the child down with medication or something to drink, and DO NOT give them a bath.

As a child wakes up, they may yell, seem disoriented, or be sleepy. There isn't necessarily a link between seizure severity and temperature. Many children are up and moving about within one to two hours after having a febrile seizure. Regardless of how short they are or how well your child behaves after one, all febrile seizures that occur for the first time should be evaluated by a doctor.

Seizures

Seizures may be caused by erratic electrical activity in the brain. There are numerous kinds of seizures, and some have relatively mild symptoms. Seizures are caused by aberrant activity on both sides of the brain, while focal or partial seizures are caused by abnormal activity in just one region of the brain. Most seizures last 30 seconds to two minutes and have no long-term harmful consequences. Seizures that last longer than five minutes, occur in succession, or during which a person does not awaken should be considered a medical emergency. Seizures may be caused by a variety of disorders, medicines, high fevers, head trauma, and other illnesses and treatments. Epilepsy is a neurological condition that causes recurring seizures in humans.

VITAL!

First Aid Treatment for Seizures

If you see someone having a seizure, do the following steps:

1. Place the person gently down. Put a folded jacket or pillow under her head and examine the soft surface for any medical identification.
2. By tilting the person's head to one side rather than restraining them, you can keep the airway open and protect it in case of vomiting.

3. Remove any spectacles, loosen ties, shirt collars, and clothing.
4. When a person regains consciousness, comfort them.

To determine if a hospital checkup is needed for any single seizures lasting less than five minutes, ask the individual whether there is any known medical history of the seizure. If there are many seizures, if they last longer than five minutes, or if the individual is pregnant, injured, or diabetic, call 911.

Fainting

Fainting, a brief loss of awareness and muscle control, leads you to lose your equilibrium. This sudden decrease in blood pressure, which reduces blood supply to the brain, is the most prevalent cause of fainting. Some of the reasons that might cause fainting include heat and dehydration, mental stress, rising up too quickly from a sitting position, some medicines, a drop in blood sugar (hypoglycemia), and heart difficulties.

VITAL!

The most frequent cause of fainting is vasovagal syncope, which is caused by a stimulus that induces an overreaction in the part of our nervous system that governs involuntary biological functions such as heart rate and blood flow. This response lowers blood pressure and heart rate, reducing blood supply to the brain and causing fainting, which may last from a few seconds to a few minutes. Common causes of vasovagal syncope include bowel movements, standing for lengthy periods of time, dehydration, witnessing blood, coughing, peeing, and feeling emotional distress. Nonetheless, there are situations when there is no evident cause.

First Aid Treatment for Fainting

If you ever feel dizzy, you should lie down or sit with your head between your knees. If you see someone fainting, you should:

1. If possible, place the individual on her back with her legs elevated over her heart to restore blood flow to the brain.
2. If the individual has not responded within one minute, contact 911.
3. Check for ABCs, start CPR if required, and watch for vomiting.

Sore Throat

Sore throats are usually caused by viruses that cause colds or other upper respiratory infections, or by bacteria such as strep throat. Sore throats may also be caused by chemicals in cigarette smoke, a scrape from anything going down your throat the wrong way, allergies, postnasal drip, and, in extreme cases, cancer. Symptoms of a sore throat often include fever, headache, nausea, and malaise because they are caused by either a viral or bacterial infection. A sore throat is characterized by pus on the surface of the tonsils, redness at the back of the throat, sensitive neck glands (inflamed lymph nodes), drooling and spitting due to throat pain, problems breathing, and small red blisters in the oral cavity.

First Aid Treatment for Sore Throat

The primary goal of treating a sore throat is to alleviate pain. There are many ways for doing so:

1. Gargle with warm salt water.
2. Take nonsteroidal anti-inflammatory drugs (NSAIDs) such as ibuprofen, naproxen, and aspirin (only if you're above the age of 16).
3. Consume enough liquids to keep hydrated; fevers frequently increase this requirement, but painful swallowing may cause fluid intake to decrease.

You may be able to drink more fluids if you use pain relievers. Caffeine is very dehydrating and should be avoided. Keeping a respectful distance from ill individuals throughout the cold and flu seasons may help you avoid viral ailments like a sore throat.

If you have a severe sore throat with minimal coughing, a temperature exceeding 101°F maintained with headache, stomach discomfort, or vomiting, or if you have signs of dehydration such as dry mouth, sunken eyes, excessive weakness, or reduced urine output, see a doctor immediately once. If your pain is severe enough that over-the-counter medications aren't helping you sleep, you should see a doctor. Go to the ER. If swallowing causes drooling, you're having difficulty breathing, or you're displaying signs of severe dehydration.

Croup

Croup, a kind of laryngitis, causes a seal-bark cough and breathing difficulty in youngsters due to enlargement of the voice box (larynx) and windpipe (tra- chea). Croup is most commonly caused by a virus, but it can also be caused by allergies, bacteria, or inhaled irritants. Although children of any age can get croup, it most commonly affects those aged six months to three years. Croup is most frequent between the months of October and March. The vast majority of cases today are not severe, but in severe cases, hospitalization may be required.

Croup symptoms include a very deep, seal-bark-like cough that is generally worst at night after many days of cOld symptoms. A child suffering with croup may have difficulty breathing, make a high-pitched squawking or crowing sound when breathing in, and have a low fever. The worst of croup usually comes during the first two or three nights and lasts around a week. The measles, Hemophilus influenzae (Hib), and diphtheria immunizations protect children against the most dangerous types of croup.

First Aid Treatment for Croup

During croup, humid and cool air helps to reduce airway swelling. At home, you can do the following:

1. After turning on the hot water in the shower or bathtub, shut the door.

2. Take your child into the bathroom once it is steamy and spend fifteen to twenty minutes with him there while the door is shut.
3. You can also take your child outside into the chilly nighttime air while they are dressed warmly.

Your child should stand up straight or sit upright to breathe more easily. The steam therapy may be beneficial, but it will not completely cure the cough, so you may need to repeat this procedure throughout the night whenever your child coughs. Additionally, you can also:

- Use a cool-mist humidifier in the room where your child sleeps. Humidifiers must be cleaned on a regular basis using a bleach and water solution to prevent mold and germ growth.
- Check that your child is drinking enough water.
- For fever, the appropriate quantity of acetaminophen or ibuprofen should be used. Never give your child aspirin or cough medicine; this will not help throat swelling and may make coughing up mucus more difficult.

If your child does not feel any better after breathing in steam and cold air, contact your doctor as soon as possible. Oral steroids were given to her to help with edema and breathing. If you suspect your child has croup, contact your doctor immediately because severe cases can lead to serious respiratory problems. Apart from coughing, hard breathing at rest may indicate a substantial, maybe deadly, throat enlargement. If your child is having problems breathing, drooling, or her lips or skin are turning blue, call 911 straight immediately.

Black Eyes

The most common cause of black eyes is blunt or blow damage to the eye or nose, which frequently results in swelling of one or both eyes and fluid accumulation in the thin, sensitive tissues of the eyelids because of the nasal injury. Facelifts, jaw surgery, head traumas, or nose surgery can all result in black eyes. The term "raccoon eyes" refers to eyes that are black, blue, and swollen. (Racoon eyes are also a sign of a particular kind of skull fracture; thus, any racoon eyes that are not the consequence of ocular trauma should be checked for a skull fracture.) Black eyes are characterized by discomfort, bruising, and swelling. Swelling and discoloration may be mild at first, with the skin becoming slightly flushed and darkening over time. When the area heals, the skin around the eye may become a dark purple, yellOw, green, or black hue; however, this coloring diminishes within a few days as the swelling goes down. A black eye may cause temporary reduced vision or difficulty opening the eye due to swelling, although chronic, serious visual impairments are unlikely. A black eye may be accompanied by a headache if the injury was caused by a blow to the head or face. Double vision, loss of sight, loss of consciousness, loss of ability to move the eye, blood or clear fluid coming from the nose or ears, blood on the surface of the eye, and a persistent headache are all serious symptoms to watch for and report to your doctor.

First Aid Treatment for Black Eyes

The following are examples of black eye first aid:

1. Use ice packs as soon as possible after the injury to help relieve pain and swelling.
2. Try to get as much sleep as possible.
3. Elevate the head of your bed while sleeping.

Use the packs for twenty minutes every hour for the first twenty-four hours. Never apply ice directly to the skin or any other area of the body; always carefully wrap the ice. A cloth-wrapped bag of frozen vegetables may also be used.

When the eye has healed, avoid doing anything that might cause more injury to the area. While most black eyes heal without complications, you should still see an ophthalmologist to ensure that your eye has not been seriously damaged. If any of the following apply, contact your doctor immediately:

- Vision changes
- The severe pain continues.
- The swelling has nothing to do with an injury.
- Fever, redness, and or pus-like discharge are signs of infection.
- You are unsure about the treatment plan or are concerned about any symptoms.

- You experience change in your behavior.
- The swelling does not start to go down after a few days.
- You have swelling around your eye caused by a bee sting.

Proceed to the emergency room or immediately consult with the doctor for any of the following listed below:

- Vision changes or loss of vision
- Inability to move your eye.
- You suspect that something has pierced your eye or is lodged within your eyeball.
- There is blood in your eye.
- Your eye seems to be distorted or to be streaming with fluid.
- Any wounds or lacerations to your head, face, or eyes

If you experience any of the following signs of a significant head or facial injury, you should seek medical attention immediately:

- Broken teeth or bones
- Vomiting after sustaining an injury
- You are unable to walk following your injury.
- Clear bloody fluids are escaping from your nose and ears.
- You're taking blood thinners.
- You have a family history of hemorrhagic diseases such as hemophilia.

Broken Nose

A broken nose is a crack or fracture of the bone component of the nose caused by trauma or a blow to the face or nose as a result of incidents such as sports injuries, personal disputes, domestic abuse, or motor vehicle accidents. A broken nose is distinguished by tenderness when touched, swelling of the face or nose, bruising of the nose or black eyes, a deformed or crooked nose, nosebleeds, a crunching or crackling sound or sensation when touching the nose that sounds like rubbing hair between two fingers, as well as pain and difficulty exhaling through the nostrils.

First Aid Treatment for Broken Nose

If you believe you have a broken nose, do the following steps:

1. Applying an ice pack to the nose right away can help to reduce discomfort and swelling. Repeat several times throughout the day and for one to two days after the accident. Always take breaks between cold-pack applications and avoid touching the skin directly with the ice.
2. To relieve pain, take acetaminophen or ibuprofen as directed. Aspirin should be avoided because it may increase the risk of bleeding and edema.
3. OTC nasal decongestants may help you breathe through your nose.

4. Sleep with your bed's head elevated to reduce nasal swelling.

A doctor should be contacted if:

- The discomfort or swelling has not subsided after three days.
- Your nose appears to be crooked.
- You can't breathe through your nose as the swelling goes down.
- You've got a fever.
- You start getting nosebleeds on a regular basis.
- You believe you have been injured and require medical treatment.

If you suspect any of the following, go to the emergency room immediately:

- You're bleeding and having trouble stopping it.
- You have clear fluids coming out from your nose.
- You have any additional facial or bodily injuries.
- You got knocked out.
- You have excruciating headaches that aren't relieved by OTC medications.
- You frequently vomit.
- Your vision has changed or deteriorated.
- You experience any neck pain.
- You have tingling, numbness, or weakness in your arms.
- Your nose is in agony.

Nosebleed

Nosebleeds are often spectacular and terrifying, but they are usually not dangerous and can be treated quickly. The two types of nosebleeds are distinguished by whether the bleeding originates in the front (anterior), which accounts for 90% of all nosebleeds, or in the back (posterior) (poste- rior). A doctor can treat minor anterior nosebleeds at home. Because posterior nosebleeds are more complicated and common in the elderly, they are often treated by an ear, nose, and throat specialist. Most people will experience a nosebleed at some point in their lives, but they are more common in children and adults aged two to eight and fifty to eighty. Nosebleeds are common in dry, cold climates, especially during the winter.

Most nosebleeds are caused by one or more identified factors, such as allergies, blunt nasal trauma, internal nasal trauma from things like nose picking or discomfort from long-term opiate use, and dry nasal passageways from dry, stale air. Nosebleeds can also be a sign of a more serious condition, such as a blood clotting disorder, blood-thinning medications, aspirin use, liver disease, obstructed blood vessels, or nasal cancer. While it is unlikely to be the only cause, high blood pressure may contribute to nosebleeds.

Most of the time, you will only have bleeding from one nostril, but if the bleeding is severe, it may flow into the space between the two nostrils within the nose and into the other nostril, resulting in bleeding on both sides. Blood may also swallow from the back of the throat and enter the mouth, causing you to have blood in your mouth or even vomit blood.

First Aid Treatment for Nosebleed

If you develop a nosebleed, follow these steps:

1. Maintain your cool by sitting up straight and tilting your head forward. If you tilt your head back, blood will flow down your neck, causing you to vomit and swallow the blood.
2. Pinch your nostrils together for 10 minutes with your thumb and forefinger. If the bleeding does not stop after ten minutes, repeat the procedure.
3. To avoid vomiting, DO NOT swallow any blood; instead, spit it out.

Avoid any further aggravating factors for the next twenty-four hours after the bleeding has stopped, such as sneezing or nasal bleeding.

Ice packs are ineffective and should not be used. Use a humidifier or vaporizer to add moisture to the air in your home if it tends to be dry, as it does for the majority of people in the winter, as well as nasal gel and saline nasal spray to keep your nose from drying out. Consult your doctor:

- Any recurring nosebleed episodes
- If you have nosebleeds in addition to other types of bleeding, such as blood in the urine or stool, consult your doctor.
- If you bruise easily.

- If you are taking any blood thinners.
- If you have any underlying conditions that could impair your ability to clot blood, such as liver or renal disease or hemophilia.
- If you are currently undergoing or have recently completed chemotherapy,

Motion Sickness

Motion sickness occurs when the signals from the inner ears, eyes, muscles, and joints to the brain DO NOT match. When traveling by car, train, aircraft, boat, or ship, you may experience motion sickness, also known as airsickness, carsickness, or seasickness. Motion sickness causes dizziness, fatigue, and nausea, which often leads to vomiting. Others only get motion sickness when traveling by boat or plane in extremely turbulent conditions, but some people are genetically predisposed to it, and it has also been linked to migraines.

First Aid Treatment for Motion Sickness

There are several options for treating motion sickness.

1. The best way to avoid motion sickness is to sit inside a large ship, facing forward, and looking out a window of a ship or aircraft.
2. For short-term journeys, the OTC drugs meclizine, also known as Dramamine, and bonine, which can also be used for intermittent symptoms, are beneficial.

3. Transderm- Scop, a prescription drug, is available as a patch that can be worn behind the ear for up to three days at a time while traveling.

Side effects of these drugs include drowsiness, sleepiness, and dry mouth. DO NOT use motion sickness medication if you have glaucoma or a urinary obstruction.

High Blood Pressure (Hypertension)

Blood pressure is influenced by two factors: the volume of blood pumped by your heart and the stiffness of your arteries against blood flow. Even with very high blood pressure—or even dangerously high blood pressure—you may not have symptoms, but some people with extremely high blood pressure may experience dull headaches, vertigo, or frequent nosebleeds.

While men are more likely than women to have high blood pressure, women frequently develop high blood pressure after menopause. African-Americans in the United States suffer from hypertension, which is frequently associated with serious complications such as heart attack and stroke.

First Aid Treatment for Hypertension

While hypertension is genetically predisposed, you can control other risk factors by increasing your level of physical activity, which benefits both your heart and your waistline. To treat and control high blood pressure, the following dietary changes and prescription drugs are used:

- Stop smoking and limit your alcohol consumption to two drinks each day.
- Lose weight to maintain a healthy weight.
- Get some exercise on a regular basis.
- Salt consumption should be reduced.
- Take your medications as prescribed.

The American Heart Association recommends at least thirty minutes of exercise every other day for heart health, while Surgeon General recommends thirty minutes of physical activity each day for general well-being. Exercise and a healthy lifestyle can help lower blood pressure and stress. Deep breathing and meditation are two stress-reduction techniques that can help.

Panic Attacks

Panic attacks can happen anywhere, at any time—alone, with others, in public, at home, or even while you're sleeping. If you have ever experienced a panic attack, you are well aware that it is similar to a period of great terror and includes the following symptoms:

- Shortness of breath (hyperventilation)
- Trembling
- Sweating
- Rapid heart rate
- Chest pain
- Abdominal cramping
- Nausea

- Chills (hot flashes)
- A feeling of tightness in your throat
- Faintness
- Dizziness
- Headache
- Difficulty swallowing
- A sense of impending death

Those experiencing a panic attack frequently believe they are having a heart attack and go to the emergency room.

A panic attack usually starts abruptly, peaks within ten minutes, and lasts about a half hour, whereas others last longer, have different patterns, and in rare cases can last up to twenty hours. During panic attacks, you may feel exhausted and overwhelmed. Anyone who suffers from panic attacks frequently suffers from panic disorder. Panic attacks can be managed or prevented with medication, counseling, and relaxation techniques. They can also be treated extremely effectively. Men have panic attacks less frequently than women.

First Aid Treatment for Panic Attacks

Stress-related symptoms and signs such as headaches, anxiety, high blood pressure, difficulty falling asleep, hyperventilation, and clenching or grinding of teeth can be reduced with relaxation techniques such as meditation, muscle relaxation, relaxed breathing, and guided imagery (visualization). Try concentrating on relaxing your body by performing the following actions:

1. Sit or lie down in a comfortable position, keep your eyes closed.
2. Allow your jaw to drop and your eyes to become heavy and relaxed, but not clenched.
3. Begin with your toes and gradually work your way up to your neck, head, arms, hands, fingers, buttocks, and legs. Concentrate on each component separately, relaxing each region before moving on to the next.
4. Tighten the muscles in each section of your body in the same order, holding for five counts before releasing and moving on to the next section.

Continue tensing and relaxing your face, shoulders, arms, legs, and buttocks muscles. While practicing relaxation, don't think about anything except how calm and at ease you feel, how heavy and warm your hands are (or, if you prefer, how cool they are), how peacefully your heart is beating, and how perfectly at peace you feel while taking deep, slow breaths.

Consider going somewhere you enjoy after you've rested. After five or ten minutes, you may gradually awaken. Use this strategy frequently. once per day or whenever you feel like you have some control over your stress. In addition to our stress-reduction strategies, it is critical to get enough sleep, avoid coffee, and maintain a regular exercise routine. If your panic attacks are recurring and you worry about them frequently for a month or longer, you may have a panic disorder and should see a doctor if you feel you need to change your behavior (for example, by avoiding places or circumstances where you've previously had an attack).

CONCLUSION

This book aims to provide you with the knowledge to keep yourself and others safe when traveling off the grid and away from help. Nobody wants to think about having to deal with an emergency, yet crises happen at the worst conceivable moments, and if you aren't prepared, disaster may hit your organization. You owe it to yourself and others to understand crisis management and human body care.

Humans are both incredibly resilient and extremely vulnerable. A person might be struck down by a slew of complaints, and chronic discomfort can result from the least reasons. Knowing how to manage diseases and injuries effectively and address both the source and symptoms is critical for grid survival. You'll have to deal with infections, wounds, shattered bones, and the trauma that comes with them, and you'll need to keep your calm to do it effectively. At such times, there is no need to panic.

We've addressed all of the possible scenarios, both small and large. When organizing a trip, it's critical to spend some time ahead of time examining potential hazards, the health of your party members, and the equipment you'll need. Consider allergies, pre-existing ailments, the environment in which you will be working, and the climate. Consider worst-case situations and how you can guarantee that everyone survives, as well as how you may prepare your party members for calamities.

Remember that the responsibility for first aid and emergency preparation should never be placed solely on one person. All adults (and children as soon as they are old enough) should accept responsibility and understand the fundamentals of first aid. Don't be hesitant to talk to the kids in the group about what to do if something goes wrong; even though you intend to be there, you might not be able to help them. A kid has the right to know how to respond appropriately to a situation, and even young children may be taught the value and usefulness of basic first aid.

Make sure you have strategies in place for natural disasters, meals, and unexpected weather changes. Even if you don't plan to deal with these extremes, your kit should always have supplies that will help you live in severe cold or extreme heat (depending on where you are). Ensure that all party members have access to the necessary materials, and consider incorporating instruction pamphlets, diagrams, and what-to-do documents in the kit so that those who are less prepared may still cope with crises.

Restock your first aid box regularly, and continually evaluate whether your approach to first aid is valid and effective. It never hurts to go over the fundamentals, especially if someone quits or joins your group. Everyone should own one.

set practices that they can follow, and a strong understanding of any health issues that others have (particularly allergies) so that they can work with them rather than against them.

Brushing first aid under the carpet and forgetting about it is easy since we aren't compelled to think about it - until the worst comes and you're stranded without necessary equipment or know-how because no one planned ahead of time. This is not a scenario you want to be in when the emergency services are far away. Don't let yourself or the people you're traveling with become victims of inaction; be prepared and equipped. You never know when you're going to need it.

You should now have a decent idea of potential circumstances and how to prepare for them. This is best complemented with hands-on instruction from experts, therefore plan to attend some first aid classes as soon as possible (with other group members if feasible). If this isn't possible, at least practice the fundamentals with other members of your party utilizing internet videos and tools. There is a variety of knowledge available, and the more you learn, the more likely you will be to remain cool and behave effectively in an emergency. It's time to get ready since tomorrow may be too late for your off-grid group's health and safety.

Made in the USA
Las Vegas, NV
21 October 2023